FOAM

Sam Woodworth

Roller

EXERCISES

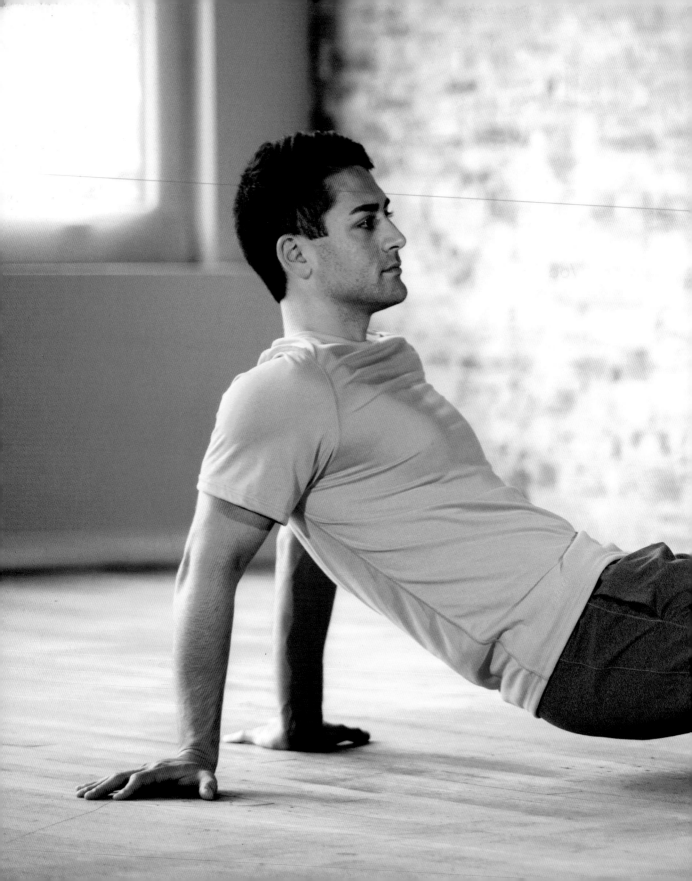

Sam Woodworth

FOAM
Roller
EXERCISES

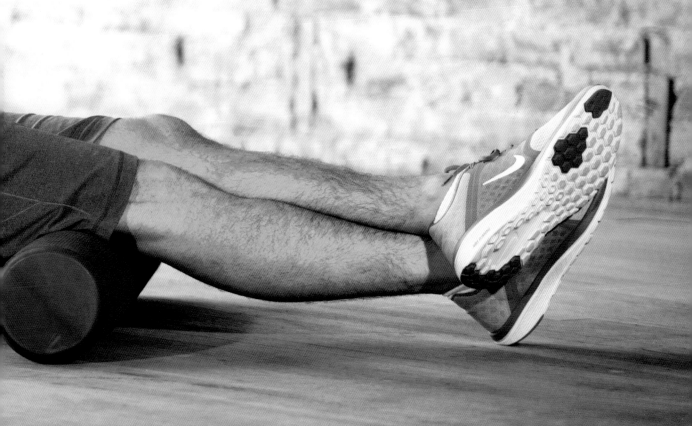

CONTENTS

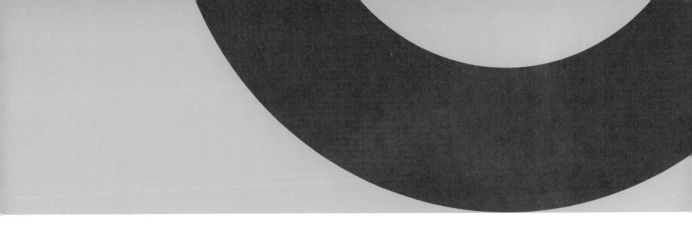

5 PAIN RELIEF PROGRAMMES

6 LIFESTYLE PROGRAMMES

7 SPORTS PROGRAMMES

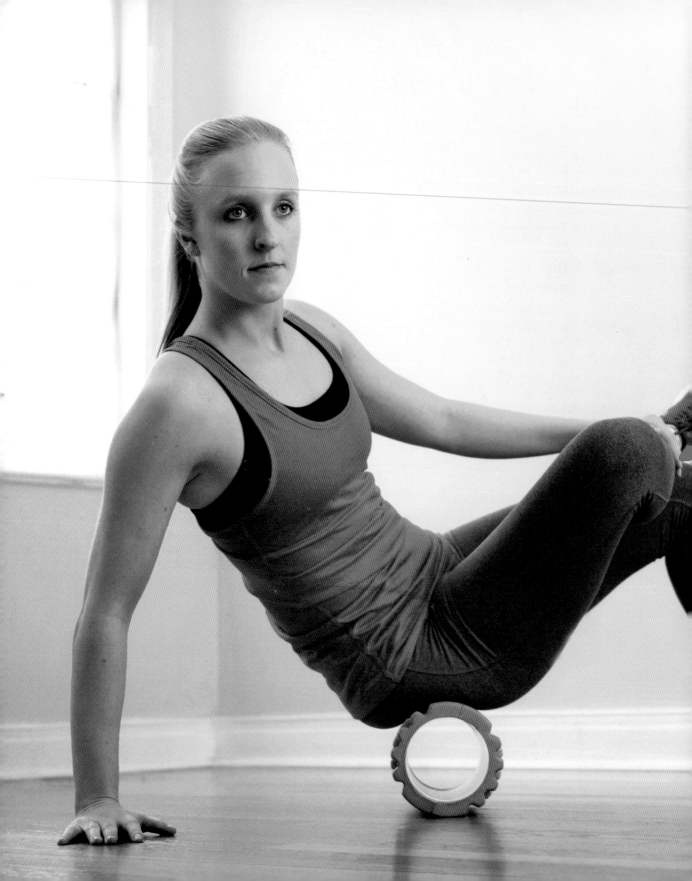

INTRODUCTION

Imagine your sense of wellness as a bucket, and optimal mobility as a full vessel, the way you're designed to work. However, if you're like most people, your movement often feels dysfunctional and strained.

Through daily lifestyle habits, you subject yourself to extremes that imbalance and weaken the muscular system – holes in the bucket, if you will. If you have poor balance, pain, limited mobility, and tightness, you'll benefit from a foam roller.

For everyone from the active and agile to the sedentary and tense, rollers and other exercise tools can counteract the negative effect of an eight-hour day sitting down, a double shift standing on your feet, or 10 miles logged as you train. Using a foam roller increases flexibility, promotes healing after injury, improves the alignment of your spine, and heightens your body awareness.

This book has 60 step-by-step exercises and 26 programmes showing you how to use rolling tools to treat the side effects of your occupational or recreational activities.

Don't allow your lifestyle to sabotage your muscles – use this book to plug the holes in your bucket as you restore your body to its healthiest, happiest, most supple state.

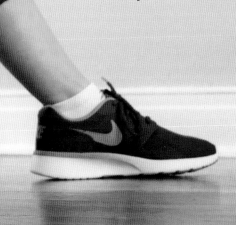

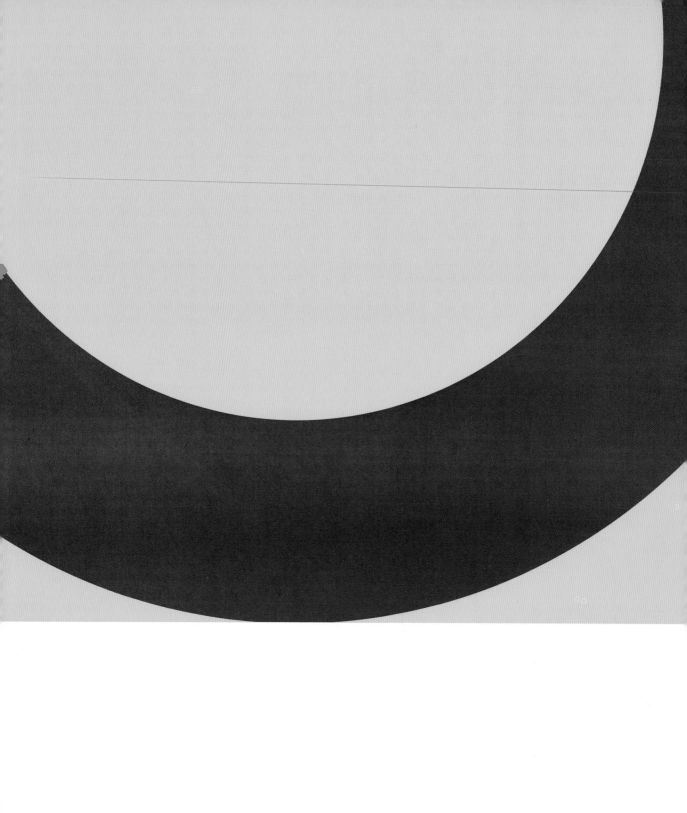

FOAM ROLLING BASICS

WHY USE A ROLLER?

The foam roller is a multi-purpose tool that can benefit just about anyone. Rollers are effective both as deep-tissue massagers and as props to build strength and bring your body into alignment.

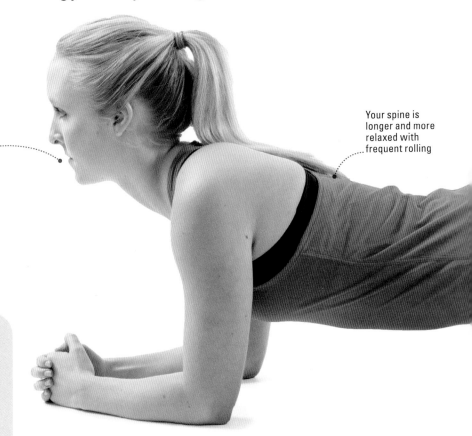

Breathing is easier when your muscles are supple

Your spine is longer and more relaxed with frequent rolling

ROLLING VS. STATIC STRETCHING

Both static stretching and foam rolling increase your range of movement. However, holding a static stretch too long and too often can reduce your muscles' ability to contract (shorten). On the other hand, foam rolling increases the flexibility of your muscles while maintaining their healthy ability to lengthen (stretch) and contract.

RELIEVE PAIN

Overworked muscles lead to aching imbalances and trigger points. Using a foam roller to massage your body's soft tissue improves circulation and alleviates pain.

IMPROVE POSTURE AND ALIGNMENT

Your muscles conform to your lifestyle, causing them to become chronically shortened or lengthened. Rolling restores muscle balance and aligns vertebrae for better posture.

MORE REASONS TO ROLL

1 It's inexpensive
Foam rolling requires little investment in equipment or gym memberships and personal trainers.

2 You can do it anywhere
Foam rollers are lightweight and easy to store, so use them at home, at the gym, or even outside.

3 You can go solo
You don't need the assistance of a coach or workout partner – just yourself and some open space.

4 It's not just for athletes
Rolling can benefit people of all abilities and lifestyles, from desk workers to stay-at-home parents.

5 It's versatile
Although it's considered a massage tool, also use it to add a challenging element to your fitness routine.

6 It helps you de-stress
Rolling away the knots and aches helps you relax at the end of a hard day, just like a deep tissue massage.

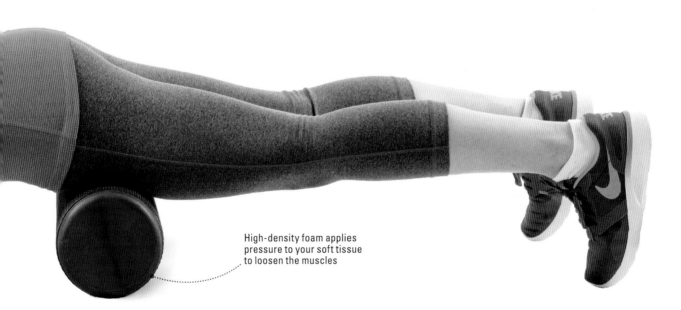

High-density foam applies pressure to your soft tissue to loosen the muscles

AID RECOVERY

The damage to muscle fibres after an injury or workout causes muscle tension. Rolling your muscles breaks up scar adhesions, reduces tightness, and accelerates healing.

INCREASE BODY AWARENESS

Underuse dulls your muscles and sensory input, but regularly using a foam roller for exercise and massage sharpens your body's sense of how it can effectively move in space.

BUILD STRENGTH

A muscular body is more functional and pain-free. Use your roller as an exercise prop to build core strength. Also challenge and build your arms and legs with massage exercises.

USING A ROLLER FOR MASSAGE

Habits and lifestyle shape your muscle use and movement, often resulting in pain and dysfunction. Using a roller and other massage tools releases tension in your body's soft tissue and restores proper movement.

WHY YOUR BODY NEEDS MASSAGE

Your occupation, fitness level, and daily habits affect your body's skeletal and neuromuscular system. These structures assimilate to your posture, so whether standing all day or sitting, your bones and soft tissues fix themselves in position. This causes muscle groups to pull on each other, with too much stress on some and not enough on others. The imbalanced system reduces your flexibility and movement quality.

MYOFASCIA AND MOVEMENT

These muscle imbalances affect your *fascia,* the flexible network of soft tissue that contains and connects every structure in your body. Muscles are specifically bound by *myofascia*. When myofascia is static, it hardens, but with mechanical stress, it is naturally more fluid. Healthy myofascia allows your muscles to slide flexibly and efficiently in your body while staying in place.

However, your myofascia thickens under stress so it can perpetuate your posture and muscle imbalances. For example, a pectoral muscle that never reaches full length develops myofascial adhesions to brace the shortened state. This causes the chest muscles to feel taut and inflexible. Hardened myofascia constricts your muscle fibres and leads to poor circulation of blood and oxygen. Restricted muscles limit your range of movement and make your body tense.

RESTORATION BY ROLLING

Massaging your muscles with a foam roller and other tools softens your myofascia so that the structures within – contracted muscle fibres – can receive oxygenated blood. This technique is called self-myofascial release (SMR). Massaging the soft tissue breaks up adhesions and returns it to a flexible state. When you practise SMR regularly, it can restore smoothness to your fascia, improve circulation, decrease pain, and increase your overall range of movement.

WHAT ARE KNOTS?

Knots (also called trigger points) are small, painful spots that form in your muscle fibres. They occur when the portion of the muscle fibre that contracts – called the *sarcomere* – becomes overworked and locked in a shortened state that restricts blood flow. Hundreds of contractions in the same spot of a muscle form a knot. Directly massaging a knot with a smaller rolling tool (such as a lacrosse or tennis ball) unlocks the sarcomeres to restore blood flow and reduce the pain.

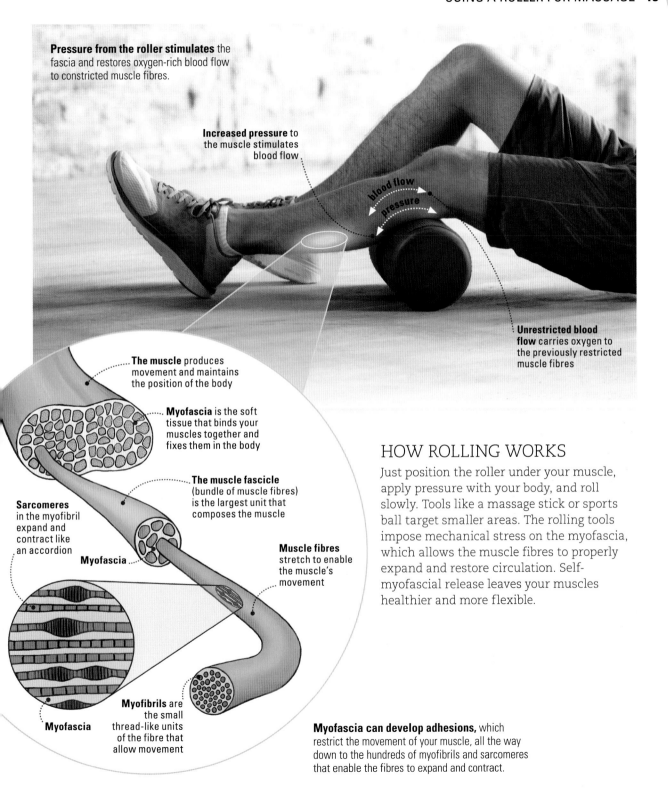

Pressure from the roller stimulates the fascia and restores oxygen-rich blood flow to constricted muscle fibres.

Increased pressure to the muscle stimulates blood flow

blood flow

pressure

Unrestricted blood flow carries oxygen to the previously restricted muscle fibres

The muscle produces movement and maintains the position of the body

Myofascia is the soft tissue that binds your muscles together and fixes them in the body

The muscle fascicle (bundle of muscle fibres) is the largest unit that composes the muscle

Sarcomeres in the myofibril expand and contract like an accordion

Myofascia

Muscle fibres stretch to enable the muscle's movement

Myofascia

Myofibrils are the small thread-like units of the fibre that allow movement

HOW ROLLING WORKS

Just position the roller under your muscle, apply pressure with your body, and roll slowly. Tools like a massage stick or sports ball target smaller areas. The rolling tools impose mechanical stress on the myofascia, which allows the muscle fibres to properly expand and restore circulation. Self-myofascial release leaves your muscles healthier and more flexible.

Myofascia can develop adhesions, which restrict the movement of your muscle, all the way down to the hundreds of myofibrils and sarcomeres that enable the fibres to expand and contract.

MORE FOAM ROLLER BENEFITS

A foam roller can also act as a prop for strength training exercises. Exercising with a roller in this way makes your movement more efficient and helps to improve your posture and balance.

BUILD CORE STRENGTH

The foam roller introduces instability to your exercises, which will intensify the engagement of your core muscles. Working out on a stable surface can eventually become too easy; by adding a foam roller, the instability requires you to engage your joints and deeper-lying muscles to help you maintain your balance. After mastering certain exercises on a stable surface, add a roller so that holding the position is more challenging. Keep your lower back static and maintain a neutral spine so that your exercises are safe and effective.

OPTIMIZE BODY AWARENESS

Whether you're minimally active or you're athletic and agile, using a roller improves body awareness, also called *proprioception*. Self-myofascial release exercises awaken and sharpen sensory input, and core-strengthening exercises require your joints and muscles to act harmoniously. Together, both types of exercise develop the signals in your muscles that provide information to your brain, asking your body to move in a particular way. You'll learn improved spatial awareness and naturally act with balance and improved reaction time.

YOGA PROP

You can use a foam roller as a prop for several yoga poses. Insert the roller into any pose where you require extra relief to your joints in an uncomfortable position. Or place the roller on the ground and use it to help you balance.

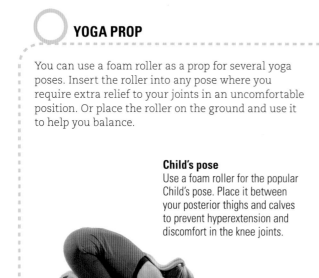

Child's pose
Use a foam roller for the popular Child's pose. Place it between your posterior thighs and calves to prevent hyperextension and discomfort in the knee joints.

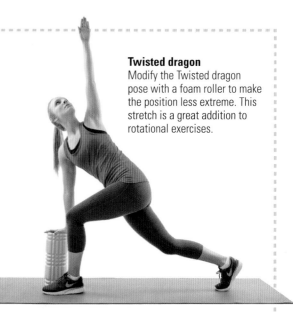

Twisted dragon
Modify the Twisted dragon pose with a foam roller to make the position less extreme. This stretch is a great addition to rotational exercises.

IMPROVE POSTURE AND ALIGNMENT

Sitting in a car or at a desk all day, looking down at a mobile phone screen, and reaching for a keyboard all deteriorate a natural and healthy posture. Foam rolling regularly will restore flexibility to your soft tissues so that your muscle groups lengthen and contract together more efficiently. Balanced and supple muscles allow your body to achieve a healthy posture and your bones to rest in pain-free alignment.

You can also use the roller as a "response" prop to strengthen weaker muscles and lock in good posture by placing the roller just beside your moving muscles during certain exercises. If the roller falls or moves excessively, you can gauge whether stronger muscles are compensating for any weaker muscles. This response method teaches your body to work more optimally, which aligns the spine and stabilizes your posture.

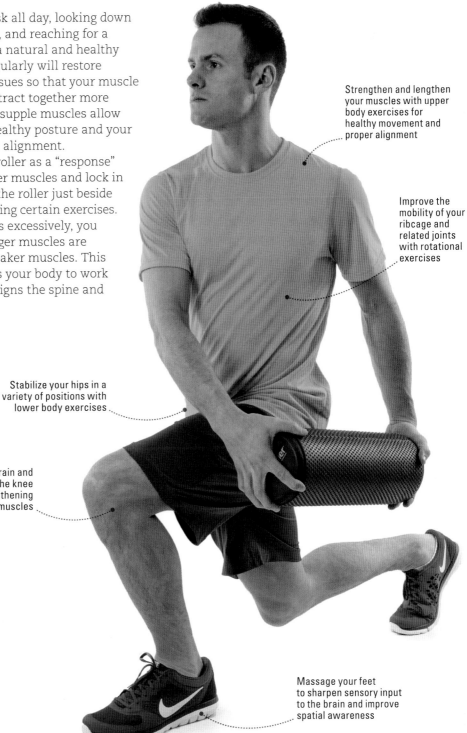

Strengthen and lengthen your muscles with upper body exercises for healthy movement and proper alignment

Improve the mobility of your ribcage and related joints with rotational exercises

Stabilize your hips in a variety of positions with lower body exercises

Minimize strain and dysfunction of the knee joints by strengthening surrounding muscles

Massage your feet to sharpen sensory input to the brain and improve spatial awareness

EFFECTIVE ROLLING

To get the most out of your rolling experience, it's important to use the roller safely by employing principles of proper breathing and positioning. It's also critical to maintain awareness of your body's response.

MONITOR YOUR BODY'S RESPONSE

Using a foam roller or other rolling tool for self-myofascial release (SMR) requires you to be attentive to your body's response. Foam rolling should elicit a "good" pain, neither excruciating nor effortless. Most exercises recommend 20 to 30 seconds of rolling, but you should listen to your body and massage only as long as the sensation feels good. A release session should leave your muscles relaxed, rejuvenated, and supple.

PAIN SCALE
Using a roller should produce pain within the 1 to 3 range. Adjust pressure so the exercises are just slightly uncomfortable.

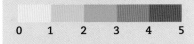

| 0 | 1 | 2 | 3 | 4 | 5 |

SMR rolling tips
- Keep breathing.
- Go slowly.
- Relax your muscles as much as possible.
- Stop rolling if it's too painful.

GET INTO POSITION

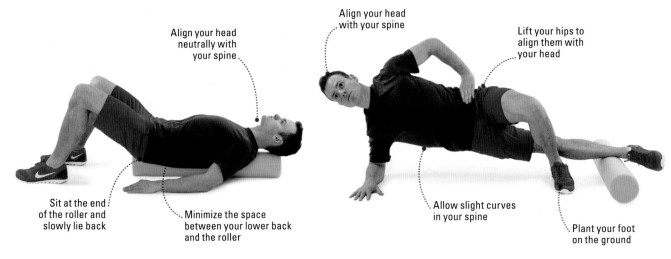

Align your head neutrally with your spine.

Align your head with your spine

Lift your hips to align them with your head

Sit at the end of the roller and slowly lie back

Minimize the space between your lower back and the roller

Allow slight curves in your spine

Plant your foot on the ground

Back-lying
Lie on the roller for exercises that target your alignment. Your lower and upper back should maintain contact with the roller throughout.

Side-lying
You'll vary this position for exercises that target muscles on the side of the body. Use your leg and forearm as supports to propel your movement.

PRACTISE CONSCIOUS BREATHING

Proper breathing is critical for maintaining a relaxed state, and only relaxed muscles are receptive to self-myofascial release. Deep, conscious breathing enhances your ability to perceive sensations and contractions in particular muscles.

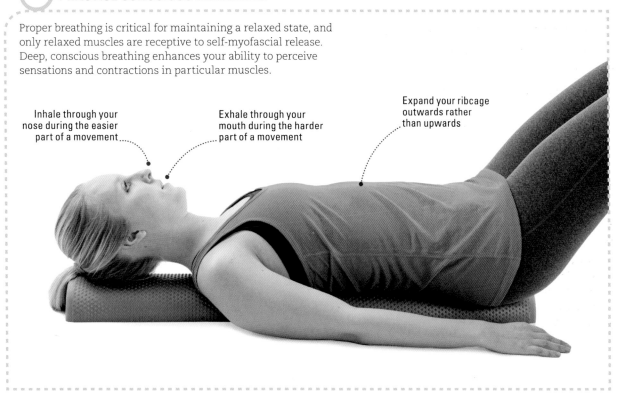

Inhale through your nose during the easier part of a movement

Exhale through your mouth during the harder part of a movement

Expand your ribcage outwards rather than upwards

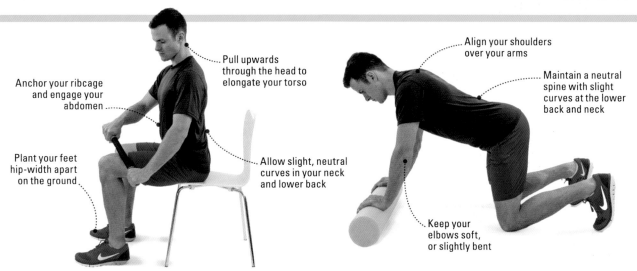

Pull upwards through the head to elongate your torso

Anchor your ribcage and engage your abdomen

Plant your feet hip-width apart on the ground

Allow slight, neutral curves in your neck and lower back

Align your shoulders over your arms

Maintain a neutral spine with slight curves at the lower back and neck

Keep your elbows soft, or slightly bent

Sitting
For exercises that require a chair, be sure to sit at the edge. To get into position, sit on your tailbone and lengthen your torso.

Kneeling or plank
Use this position to engage the abdomen for many core exercises. For effective exercises, channel pressure through your arms as they support you.

WHAT YOU NEED

The exercises in this book don't require lots of expensive or hard-to-find equipment. Choose your tools based on your degree of body awareness, level of pain perception, and overall goals.

ROLLERS

Foam rollers come in a variety of shapes, sizes, textures, and colours. Texture and density affect the intensity of your release, and the size and shape of a roller make it particularly suited for certain exercises. You'll want to select a roller that can meet a majority of your needs and goals. For basic massage and exercise when you're just starting out, it's best to keep it simple with a circular roller.

You can rest your whole back and head on these longer rollers

Circular roller

This is the most common type of roller, available in all sorts of lengths and densities. It's used for most of the exercises in this book.

Half roller

The half roller doesn't actually roll, but it's more stable than a circular roller and is a useful prop to stand on in many exercises.

Stand with the curved side to the ground to challenge your balance

TIP
When choosing a roller, consider how to maximize mechanical stress on soft tissue without exceeding your pain tolerance. Try a smooth, 92cm (36in) roller to begin with.

Textured roller

This advanced foam roller uses texture to provide points of increased pressure on your soft tissue. The extra mechanical stress elicits extra release.

Spikes and ridges deeply penetrate the fascia

◯ CHOOSING THE RIGHT ROLLER

There is no one-size-fits-all foam roller. The best roller for you is one that's comfortable, effective, and not too painful. If you can, test your roller before you buy it.

Consider these factors:

1 Shape
Choose a circular roller if you want to release large muscles groups or to perform most core and balance exercises. Use a half roller as an exercise prop if you want to modify exercises in which you're not actually rolling the foam roller.

2 Length and diameter
Consider that a longer roller is bulkier but stable and great for back exercises. A shorter roller is harder to control but more portable and best for leg exercises.

Most are 46 or 92cm (18 or 36in) long. While they're usually 15cm (6in) in diameter, a smaller diameter is great for ageing or physical therapy patients.

3 Material and density
Determine if your pain tolerance and desired level of release require a more or less dense roller. A standard roller uses high-density foam and provides moderate release, while a plastic core roller (often hollow) provides more intense release.

4 Texture
Choose texture based on your level of muscle tension. A roller with bumps and ridges adds additional points of pressure to your soft tissue, which maximizes release. A smooth roller distributes pressure, so the massage is more gentle.

OTHER TOOLS

Several exercises and modifications in this book incorporate sports balls and massage sticks. They give additional control and pressure to your exercises, which are especially important for relieving trigger points.

Sports balls
Firm sports balls are crucial for trigger point release. They provide a concentrated point of pressure for tense muscles. This book features a massage ball in the targeted release exercises.

Massage ball

Golf ball

Tennis ball

OTHER EQUIPMENT YOU MAY WANT

Yoga mat Many exercises require you to be on the ground, so a non-slip mat increases your comfort and safety.

Chair Some exercises and modifications are easier if you sit on a chair or rest your hands on it for balance.

Pillow You may want to lie on a pillow to relieve any neck tension, or place a pillow on the ground for some back-lying rotational exercises.

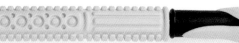

Massage stick
This piece of equipment provides more targeted release than a foam roller. Since you hold a massage stick with your hands, it's a good way to modify any exercise to make a position and movement easier.

BEFORE YOU BEGIN

Before you get started with this book, take some time
to consider what your needs are and which programmes
or exercises best suit you. With the right tools and the
right environment, you're ready to get rolling.

EVALUATE YOUR NEEDS

Everyone engages in repetitive patterns of
movement that disrupt the body's alignment and
cause muscle tension and pain. Consider your daily
habits and areas of pain, and choose the exercises
and programmes that will benefit you most.

CHOOSE A PROGRAMME

In the last three chapters of the book are 26
programmes (each 5 to 10 exercises) that tend to
particular needs. Some address work conditions,
and others athletic activities. For example, if you
play tennis, try the rotational sports programme.

HABIT AND EFFECT	REMEDY
Spending all day at a desk overworks and underuses a myriad of muscles within the legs, hips, and spine, which imbalances the whole muscular system.	**Roll the hip flexors, hamstrings, and chest area,** and strengthen your entire backside. Releasing knots may be necessary in the upper back and shoulders.
Driving more than an hour strains muscles in your upper back and shoulders and shortens the chest muscles, in addition to underworking the legs and hips.	**Release the chest muscles** to reduce tightness, and strengthen the upper back muscles to improve posture. Massage your hip flexors and quadriceps.
Looking down at a phone or tablet shortens muscles in the front of the neck and the chest and overstretches muscles in the back of the neck and upper back.	**Roll the chest, shoulders, and arms** to reduce tightness. You may also need to address trigger points of the lower arms and hands caused by holding devices.
Frequently reaching overhead overlengthens the neck and shoulder muscles and strains the lower back, which deteriorates alignment.	**Release the shoulders and upper back,** and choose exercises to lengthen and restore your spine to improve vertebral alignment.
Spending all day on your feet stiffens your hips and legs, reduces flexibility, and inflames the fascia in the bottom of the feet.	**Massage your feet** and roll the entire lower body to improve your range of motion in stiff joints. Strengthen your core and lower body muscles.
Carrying a heavy bag on your shoulder creates asymmetry in your shoulder and hip alignment and throws off your natural gait.	**Release your shoulders and core,** especially on the side where you carry the load. Perform rotational exercises to offset asymmetry.

FOAM ROLLING Q&A

How often should I use a roller?
Use a foam roller at least three times per week for the best results. There's no research that too much self-myofascial release is harmful.

How long should I spend on each exercise?
Usually 20–30 seconds provides adequate release, but roll for as long or as short as feels good.

Using a roller hurts! Am I doing it wrong?
Some discomfort is normal, but don't exceed your pain tolerance. In general, if you can't maintain comfortable breathing, reduce the pressure.

Can I create my own programme?
Yes, modify the programmes in this book or create your own to fit your lifestyle or limitations. Determine your primary need, and choose 5 to 10 exercises. For thorough release, foam roll first, then do the targeted release exercises.

What kind of results can I expect?
If you do the exercises properly and frequently, you can expect less pain, better posture, and enhanced mobility in previously restricted joints. You'll feel better after just one release session, so keep it up.

When should I use my foam roller?
Roll whenever you have time, but especially before and after a workout. Rolling before you go to bed can give you a more relaxed sleep, and rolling when you wake up primes your body for a productive day.

Who can benefit from foam rolling?
Anyone from elite athletes to desk workers can benefit from massage.

Should I do it even if I don't have any issues?
Yes! Prevention plays a critical role in maintaining your muscles, so massage regularly to keep them healthy and flexible.

 COUNTDOWN TO ROLLING

- Use your foam roller in an open space with room to fully extend your arms and legs.
- Pull back long hair and avoid thick, baggy clothing.
- Find a non-slip surface on which to do your exercises.
- Remove your shoes if you plan to stand on the roller or massage your feet.

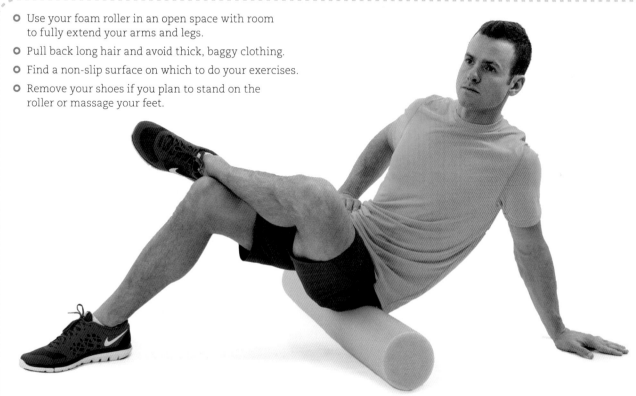

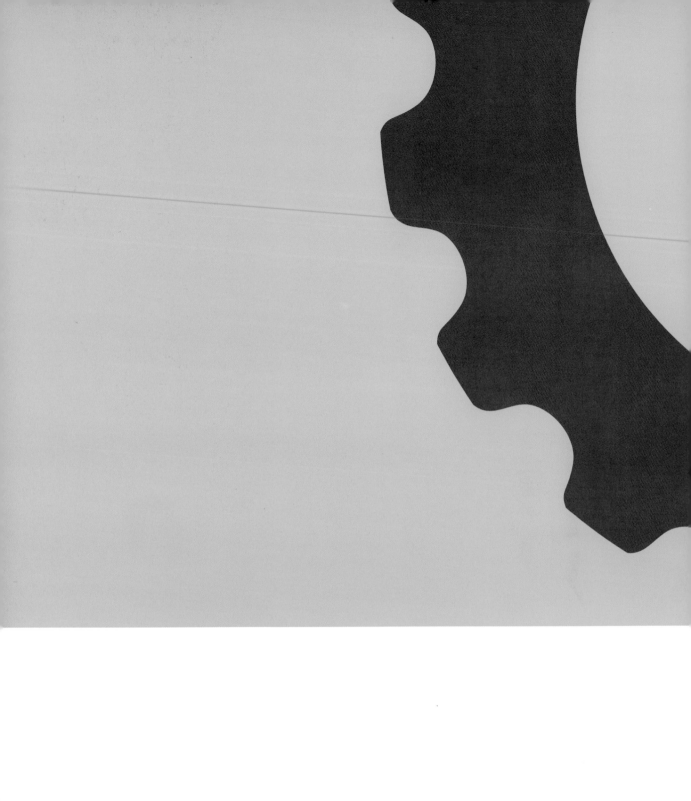

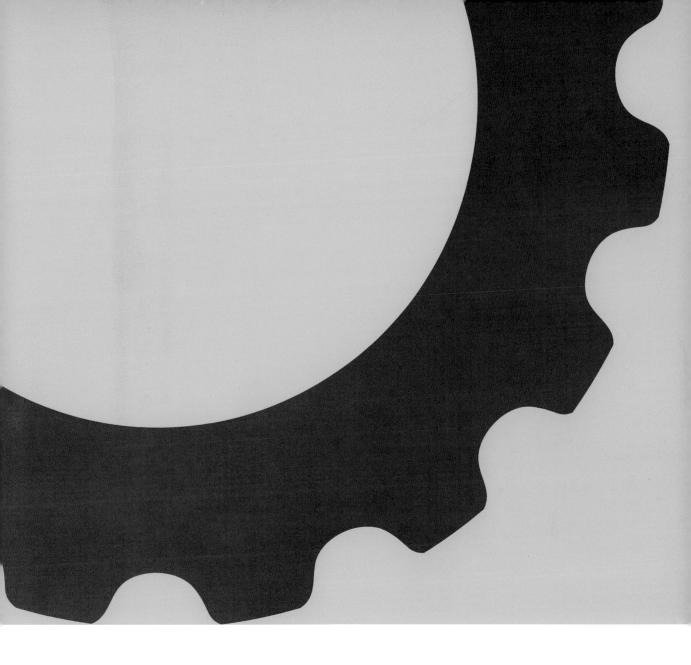

CORE
EXERCISES

PLANK PROGRESSIONS

Since crunches and sit-ups reinforce rounded posture, the plank is a great way to support an erect stance. This exercise outlines three progressions – advance your plank when you master the previous one with strength and perfect posture.

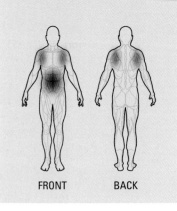

TARGETED MUSCLES

This exercise targets the obliques, the abdomen, and the shoulder blade stabilizers. Strengthening these muscles makes the body more stable and efficient.

FRONT   BACK

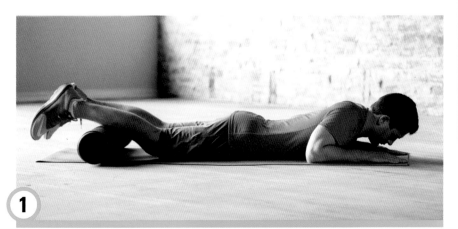

(1)

Lie on your stomach and place the foam roller beneath your shins. Put your forearms and palms flat on the ground.

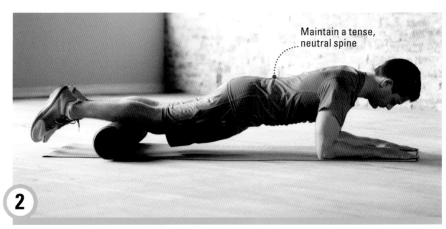

Maintain a tense, neutral spine

(2)

Lift your body off the ground by pushing through your forearms, and contract your abdomen. Hold for 1 minute.

HOW IT HELPS

Planks strengthen the core to restore posture. The spinal position is often compromised, but engaging the abdomen stabilizes the vertebral column.

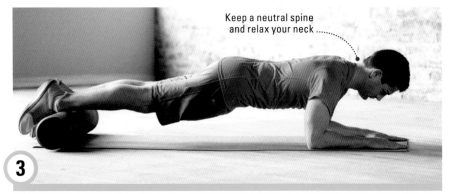

Keep a neutral spine
and relax your neck ·····

3

Progress to a more difficult plank by shifting the
roller closer to your feet. Hold for 1 minute.

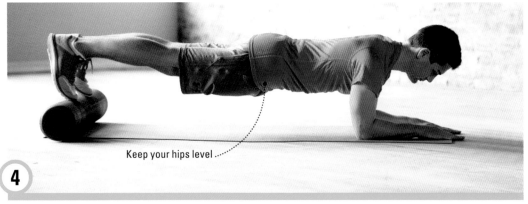

Keep your hips level ·····

4

Shift the roller down beneath your toes. Hold the
plank for 1 minute.

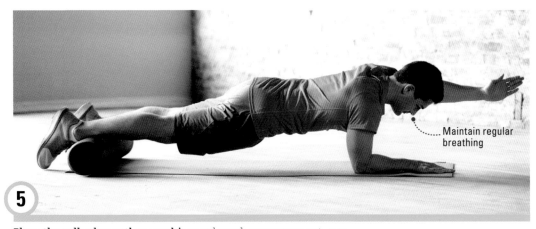

Maintain regular
breathing

5

Place the roller beneath your shins and reach your arms out, one
at a time. Alternate your reach with each arm for 1 minute.

ROLLER ROLLOUT

Lock in good posture throughout your day by doing the Roller rollout. This core-strengthening exercise produces a bigger contraction of the abdomen than a traditional sit-up, so it dramatically improves your body's ability to remain in alignment.

TARGETED MUSCLES

This exercise targets the core musculature and the *latissimus dorsi* and *teres major* muscles of the back. These influence shoulder position and spinal alignment.

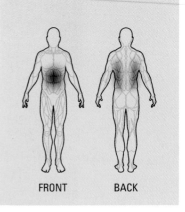

FRONT   BACK

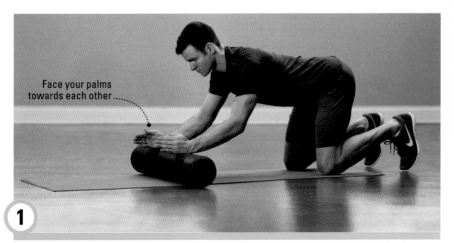

Face your palms towards each other

1

Kneel and place the foam roller in front of you. Position the sides of your hands on the roller, shoulder-width apart.

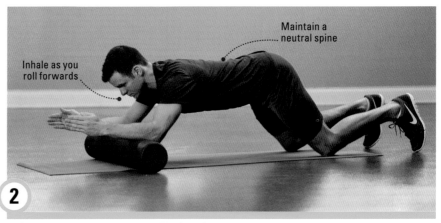

Maintain a neutral spine

Inhale as you roll forwards

2

Roll forwards from the hips, allowing the roller to glide up your hands and forearms.

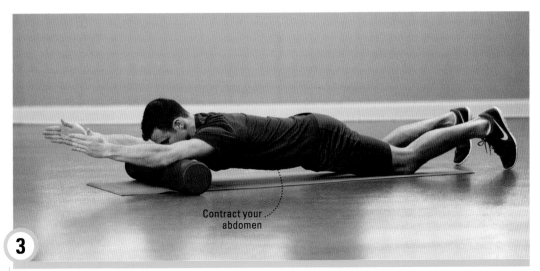

Contract your
abdomen

3

Continue to roll over the foam roller until your
arms and hips reach full extension.

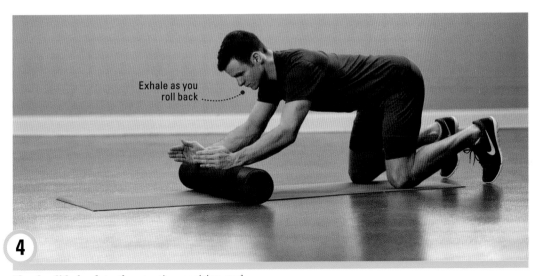

Exhale as you
roll back

4

Slowly slide back to the starting position and
repeat the exercise 15 times.

CAUTION
To avoid shoulder
or back injury, stop if
you feel any pain and
regress to a less
challenging core
exercise such as Plank
progressions.

ROLLER WALKOUT

This challenging core and shoulder exercise improves torso stability in many positions, such as standing upright and sitting. The Roller walkout translates to better posture and balance during exercise and daily activities by strengthening the core.

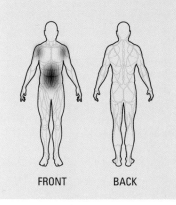
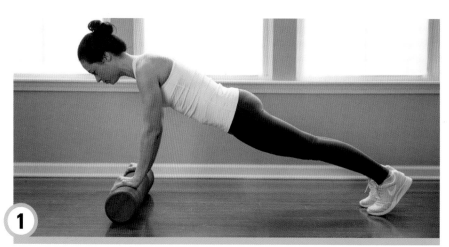

1

Place your hands shoulder-width apart on the foam roller and lift your body into a push-up position. Align your shoulders over your arms.

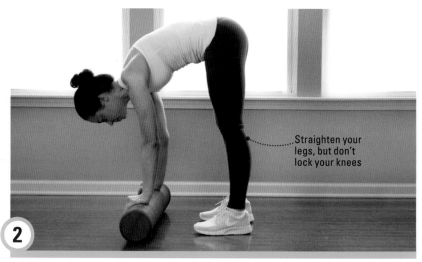

Straighten your legs, but don't lock your knees

2

Walk your feet in towards your hands, keeping your legs straight and lifting your hips until they're aligned over your feet.

TIP
To improve stability in the shoulder joints, point your middle finger up and rotate your arms inwards as you walk forwards.

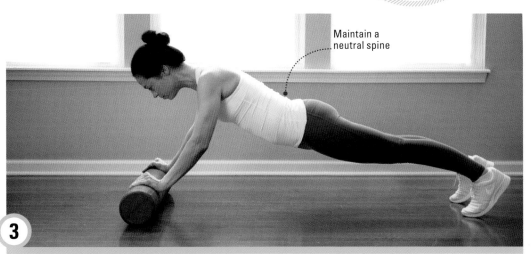

Maintain a neutral spine

3

Walk your feet back as far as possible, extending your arms, straightening your legs, and engaging your core.

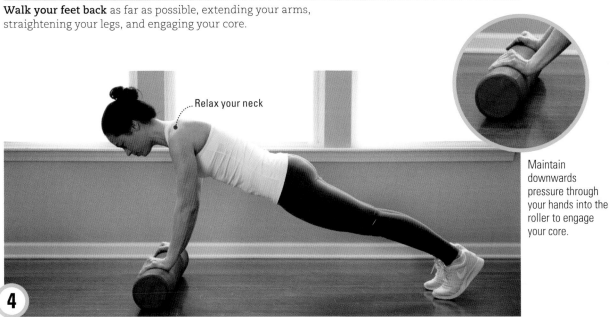

Relax your neck

Maintain downwards pressure through your hands into the roller to engage your core.

4

Walk your feet slightly forwards to return to the starting position. Repeat the exercise 10 times.

BIRD DOG REACH

Incorporating the foam roller with the Bird dog reach exercise improves your balance and tests your ability to distribute load across one hip and shoulder. It's a great way to develop spine and hip control during one-leg-stance actions such as walking.

TARGETED MUSCLES

This exercise targets the abdominals, obliques, gluteals, and deltoids, which stabilize the pelvis and torso and improve movement efficiency.

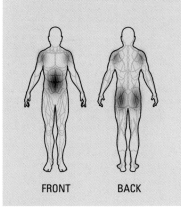

FRONT   BACK

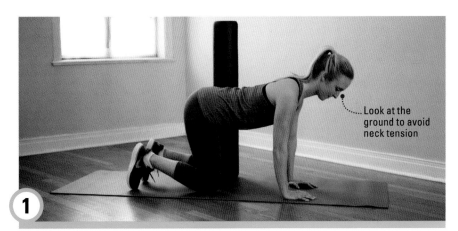

Look at the ground to avoid neck tension

1

Kneel on all fours and place the foam roller next to your left hip. Align your shoulders over your hands and your hips over your knees.

TIP
To keep excessive pressure off your wrists and to stabilize your torso, channel your weight through the supporting palm and knee.

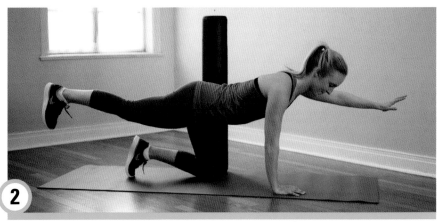

2

Reach your left arm straight out in front of you and reach your right leg straight out behind you, trying not to move the roller.

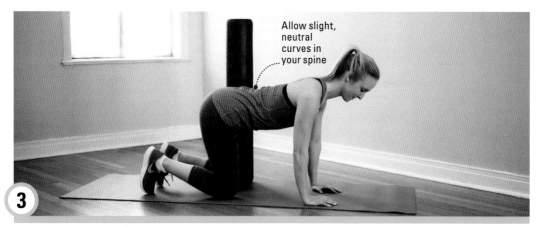

Allow slight, neutral curves in your spine

3

Return your arm and leg to the starting position, trying not to move the roller. Repeat the exercise 10 to 15 times with your left arm and right leg.

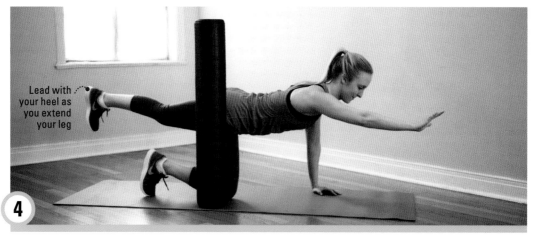

Lead with your heel as you extend your leg

4

Switch the roller to your right hip and repeat the exercise with your right arm and left leg.

MODIFICATIONS

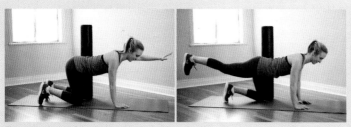

To make it easier, first move just your arm, then progress to moving just your leg.

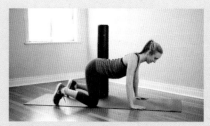

To make it harder, widen your knees and hands to challenge your core muscles.

HIP SWIVEL

For those with limited spine mobility or for rotational sport athletes, this core exercise addresses issues with the rotation of the pelvis and torso. Using the foam roller activates the hip adductors and challenges your core, integrating them for effective twisting.

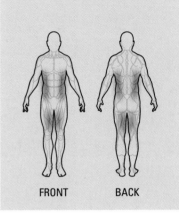
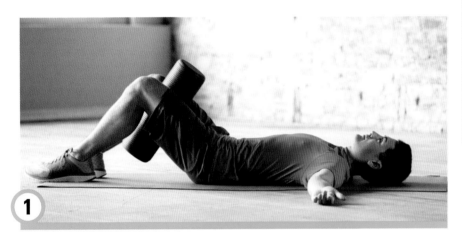

1

Lie on your back and extend your arms out from your body, palms facing up. Plant your feet on the ground and place the foam roller between your knees.

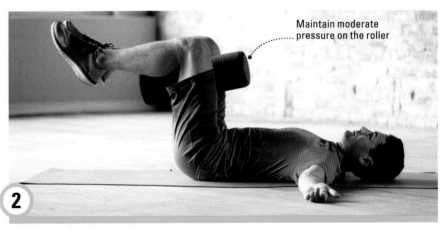

Maintain moderate pressure on the roller

2

Raise your legs, align your knees over your hips, and bend your knees to 90 degrees.

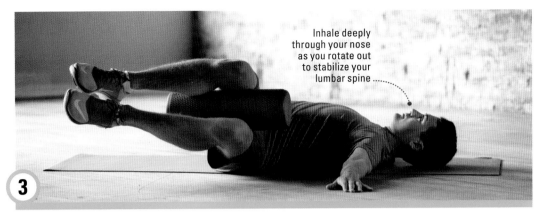

Inhale deeply
through your nose
as you rotate out
to stabilize your
lumbar spine

3

Rotate your hips and thighs to the left and rotate
your left arm. When your right shoulder begins
to lift off the ground, rotate back to the starting
position. Repeat the exercise 10 times to the left.

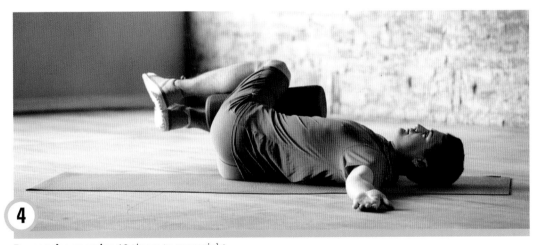

4

Repeat the exercise 10 times to your right.

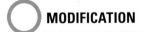 **MODIFICATION**

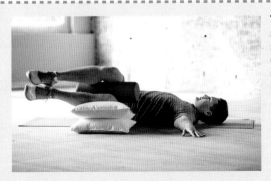

To make it easier,
stack pillows on each
side of your body to
establish easier
endpoints for your
range of movement.

TIP
For less tension in your
neck, lay your head on
a pillow. Minimal
tension in peripheral
muscles makes the
exercise safer and
more effective.

SITTING RIBCAGE ROTATION

If you sit for prolonged periods, you'll benefit from this mobility-enhancing exercise. A good range of movement in your thoracic spine limits excessive movement in the lower back. Using the roller to activate your adductors helps to stabilize the often painful area.

TARGETED MUSCLES

This exercise targets the thoracic spine, from the neck to the lower back, as well as the abdomen. These areas are responsible for bending and twisting the torso.

FRONT   BACK

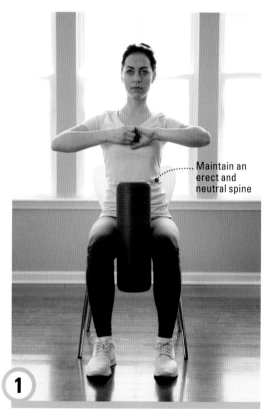

Maintain an erect and neutral spine

1

Sit on the edge of a chair and place the foam roller between your knees. Clasp your hands together and place them on your sternum. Bend your hips, knees, and ankle joints to 90 degrees.

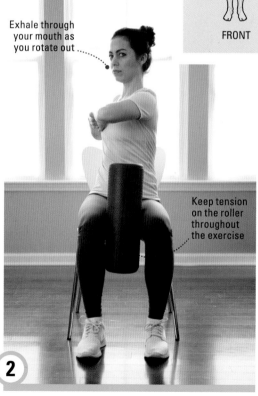

Exhale through your mouth as you rotate out

Keep tension on the roller throughout the exercise

2

Rotate your arms and torso to the right until you reach the end of your range of movement.

TIP
To fix asymmetrical alignment, do more repetitions to one side. For example, golfers or painters may have more tightness in one side than the other.

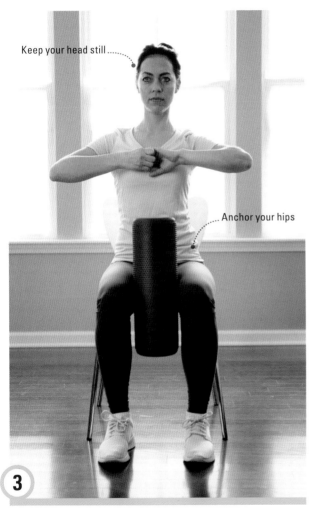

Keep your head still

Anchor your hips

3

Rotate back to the starting position and repeat the full rotation 20 times to your right side.

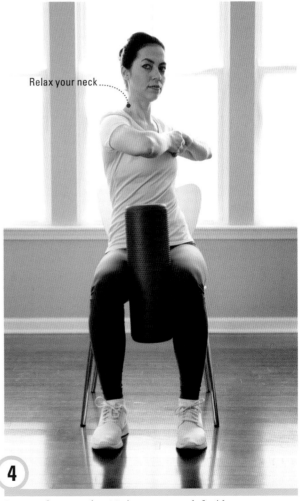

Relax your neck

4

Repeat the exercise 20 times to your left side.

HALF-KNEELING CORE ROTATION

To mimic everyday mechanical movements such as walking and running, the Half-kneeling core rotation dynamically incorporates the hips with torso rotation. By using a roller for feedback, it indicates whether hip tightness inhibits your rotational performance.

TARGETED MUSCLES

This exercise targets the core muscles, the gluteal group, and the hip adductor muscles. They help to rotate the torso from side to side while walking.

FRONT   BACK

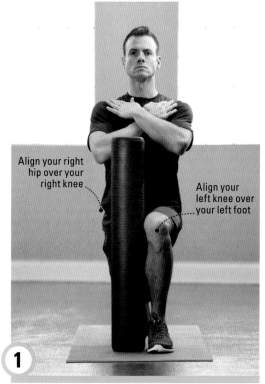

Align your right hip over your right knee

Align your left knee over your left foot

1

Kneel on your right knee and plant your left foot on the ground. Place the foam roller beside the inside of your left knee and cross your arms over your chest. Inhale to prepare for the movement.

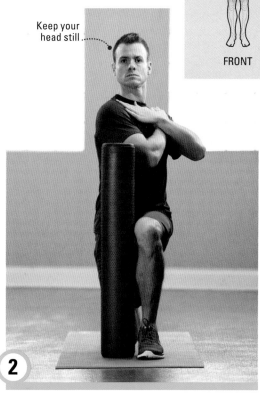

Keep your head still

2

Engage your right gluteals, exhale, and rotate your torso to the left. When you reach the end of your range of movement, rotate back to the starting position. Repeat 10 times to the left.

TIP
To improve your ability to do the rotation, also perform release exercises for your lats and gluteal group. Poor flexibility in one muscle group inhibits the other group.

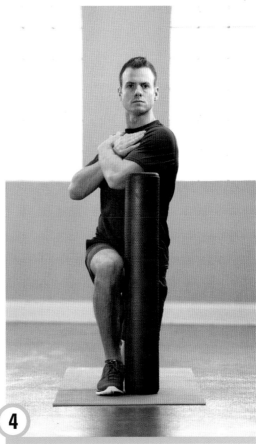

4

Repeat the rotation 10 times to the right.

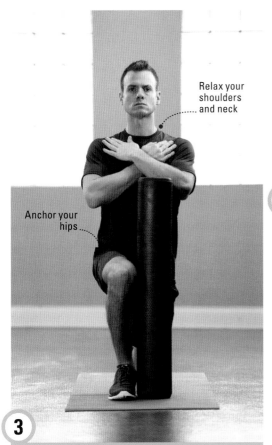

Relax your shoulders and neck

Anchor your hips

3

Kneel on your left knee, switch the roller to the inside of your right knee, and cross your arms.

MODIFICATION

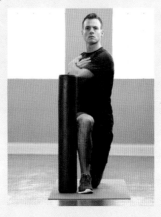

For a different type of muscle response, place the foam roller beside the outside of your support knee.

SIDE-LYING RIBCAGE ROTATION

The Side-lying ribcage rotation strengthens your ability to perform thoracic rotation (twisting of the upper and middle back) in relation to your inner thighs. It's a good intermediate challenge if you find the Half-kneeling core rotation too difficult.

TARGETED MUSCLES

This exercise targets the adductor muscle group of the inner thighs and the core muscles. These muscles control leverage for torso rotation.

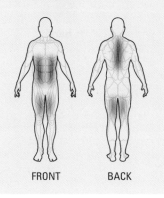

FRONT   BACK

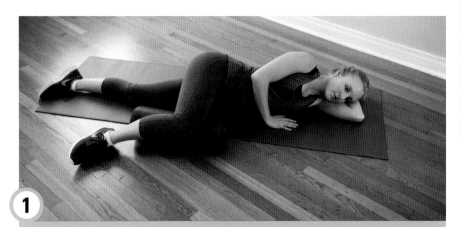

1

Lie on your left side, straighten your left leg, and bend your right knee and hip to 90 degrees. Place the foam roller beneath your right knee.

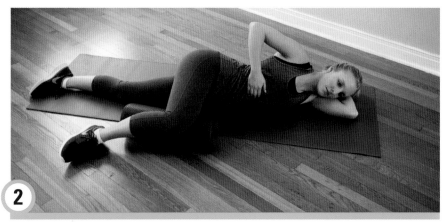

2

Grasp your ribcage with your right hand, slightly below your sternum, and inhale.

CAUTION
To avoid muscular strain, do not exceed a comfortable range of movement. Your level of mobility should determine your degree of rotation.

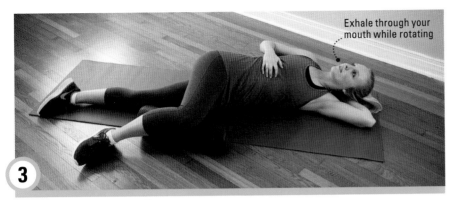

Exhale through your mouth while rotating

3

With your right hand, pull your torso back as far as possible without allowing your right knee to lift off the roller.

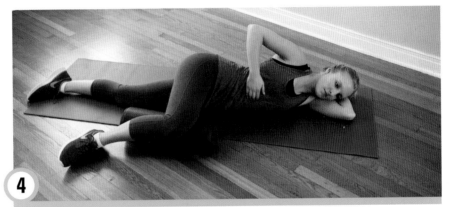

4

Slowly return to the starting position and repeat the rotation 10 times to the right.

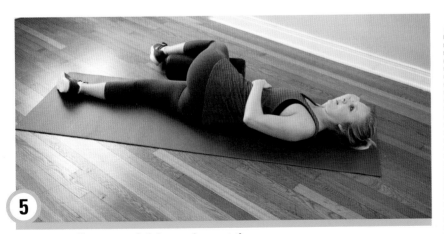

5

Move the roller to your left leg, and repeat the rotation 10 times to the left.

MODIFICATION

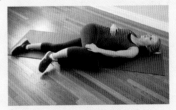

To increase pressure, use your resting arm and push your knee against the roller for a deeper rotation.

STRAIGHT-LEG RAISE

A great staple for any exercise routine, the Straight-leg raise emulates the mechanical movements of walking and running. The exercise integrates core strength with your ability to stabilize one hip while mobilizing the other, as you do in any single-leg stance.

TARGETED MUSCLES

This exercise coordinates movement of the hip flexors, obliques, and abdomen. These are essential for walking.

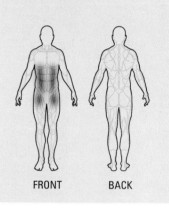

FRONT   BACK

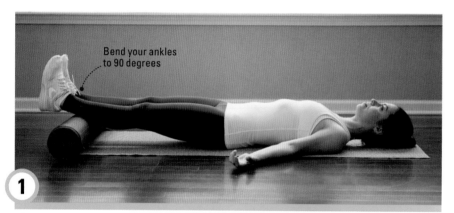

Bend your ankles to 90 degrees

1

Lie on your back, relax your arms, straighten your knees, and place your ankles side by side on the foam roller.

TIP
To take tension off your lower back, engage your core muscles. This allows better mobility in your moving leg.

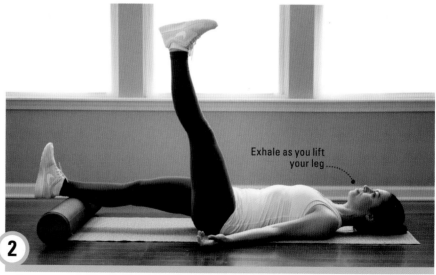

Exhale as you lift your leg

2

Raise your left leg straight up, as high as possible without pain or bending your knee. Keep your right leg fixed on the roller.

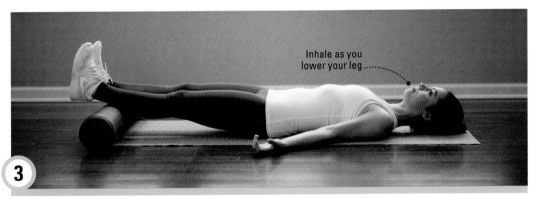

Inhale as you
lower your leg

3

Lower your left leg to the starting position and repeat
the raise 10 times with your left leg.

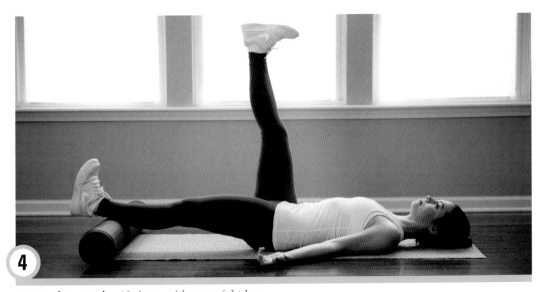

4

Repeat the exercise 10 times with your right leg.

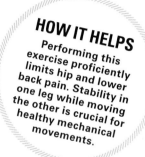

HOW IT HELPS
Performing this
exercise proficiently
limits hip and lower
back pain. Stability in
one leg while moving
the other is crucial for
healthy mechanical
movements.

MODIFICATION

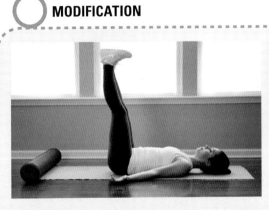

**To make it
harder,** raise
both legs, feet
flexed, and
alternate tapping
the roller with
each leg.

LOWER BODY
EXERCISES

OVERHEAD SQUAT

This more advanced exercise is an excellent full body workout to secure improved posture after a release session. It improves coordination of your muscles from your upper back to your ankles, and the arm component develops overhead mobility.

TARGETED MUSCLES

This exercise targets the lower body muscles, the core muscles, and the shoulders. The total body movement strengthens your muscular system.

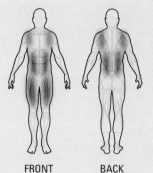

FRONT   BACK

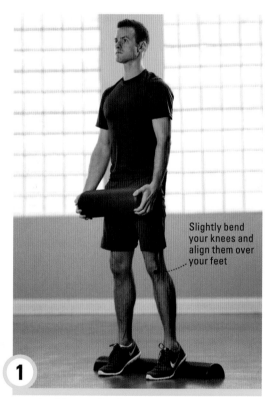

Slightly bend your knees and align them over your feet

1

Stand with your heels on the curved part of a half foam roller, slightly wider than shoulder-width apart. Hold the ends of a circular roller.

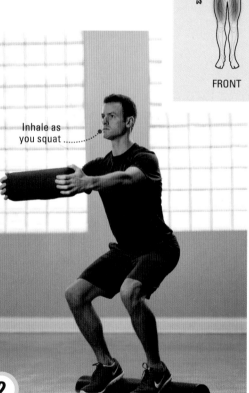

Inhale as you squat

2

Slowly bend at the hips by sitting your pelvis back and bending your knees. At the same time, begin to raise your arms.

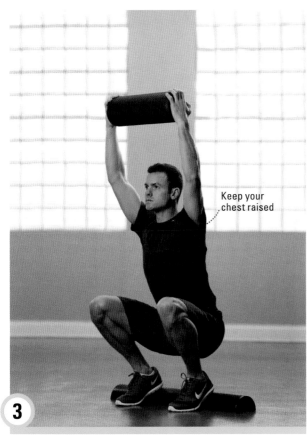

Keep your chest raised

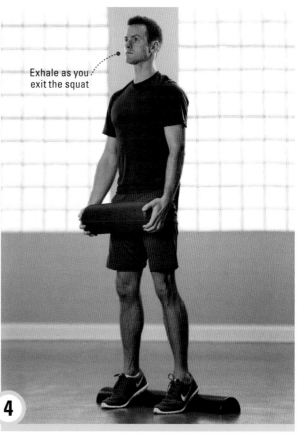

Exhale as you exit the squat

3

Squat as deeply as possible and raise your arms until they're straight overhead with your wrists aligned with or behind your head.

4

Slowly return to the starting position and repeat the exercise 15 times.

◯ MODIFICATIONS

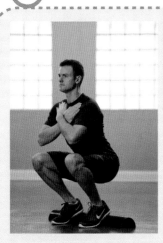

To make it easier, cross your arms over your chest if raising them is hard or painful.

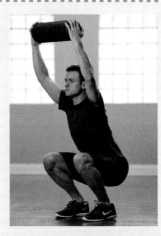

To make it harder, remove the half roller and plant your feet flat on the ground.

ROTATIONAL LUNGE

This dynamic exercise is a challenging way to improve the symmetry of your lower body and core muscles. Performing it often is great for any athletic endeavour or lifestyle, as it strengthens and balances the complex movement of several muscle groups.

TARGETED MUSCLES

This exercise targets the gluteal group, quadriceps, hamstrings, and abdomen. Coordination of these muscles is necessary for total movement efficiency.

FRONT   BACK

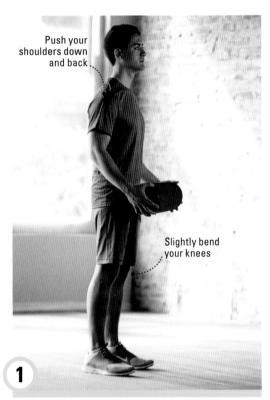

Push your shoulders down and back

Slightly bend your knees

1

Stand upright, centre your weight over your feet, and hold the ends of the foam roller.

Keep your head still

Anchor your hips as you rotate

2

Step your right foot forwards and lower your body. As you lunge, rotate your torso to the right and reach the roller around your right leg.

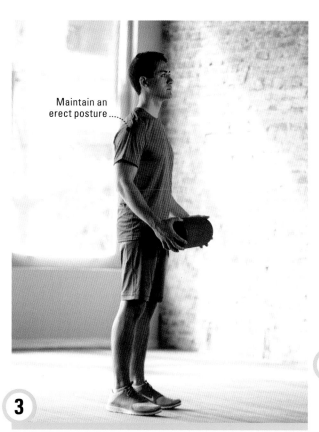

Maintain an erect posture

3

Press through your left foot, engage the gluteals, and rotate and step back to the starting position.

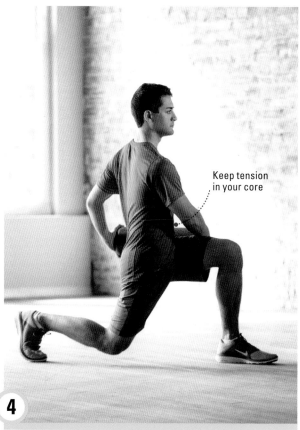

Keep tension in your core

4

Repeat the exercise to your left side. Alternate lunging on each side for a total of 20 repetitions.

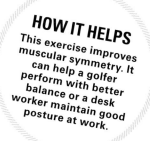

HOW IT HELPS
This exercise improves muscular symmetry. It can help a golfer perform with better balance or a desk worker maintain good posture at work.

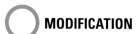 **MODIFICATION**

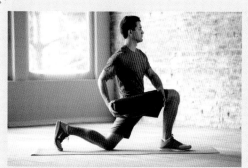

To make it easier, kneel on one knee and coil and uncoil your torso 10 times to one side, then swap your stance and repeat for the opposite side.

ADDUCTOR CHAIR SQUAT

This advanced squat is a great full body conditioner. Adding the roller minimizes the distance between your legs and makes the movement more challenging. If you want to lengthen and strengthen your body, then this exercise is a perfect workout addition.

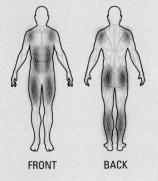

TARGETED MUSCLES

This exercises targets the deltoids in the shoulder, the abdomen, the gluteal group, the quadriceps, and the *gastrocnemius* muscles in the calves. They're important for movement efficiency and posture.

FRONT   BACK

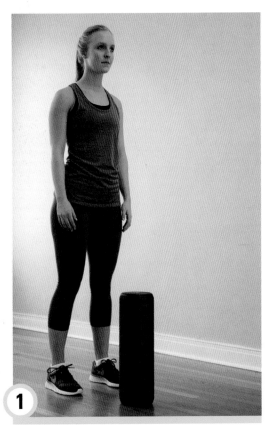

1

Stand upright with your feet shoulder-width apart and point your toes forwards.

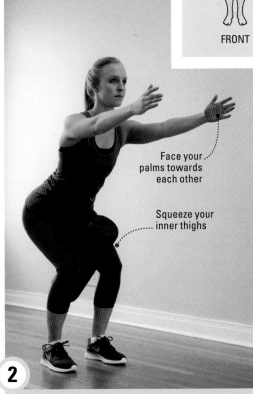

Face your palms towards each other

Squeeze your inner thighs

2

Place the foam roller between your thighs. Bend at the hips, sitting your pelvis back and bending your knees. Begin to raise your arms straight up.

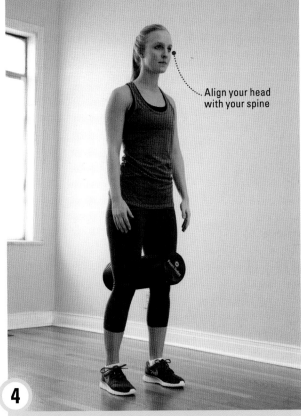

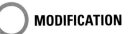

Align your head
with your spine

4

Return to the starting position by lowering your arms, contracting your gluteals, and raising your hips. Repeat the exercise 10 to 15 times.

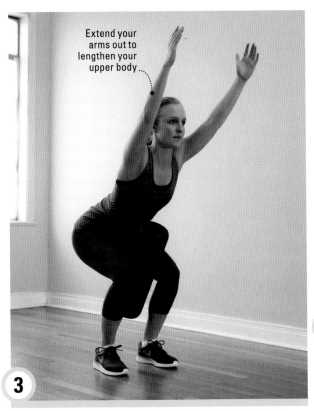

Extend your
arms out to
lengthen your
upper body

3

Squat to a comfortable depth and raise your arms until they're aligned with your back.

HOW IT HELPS
This squat balances your knee stabilizers: the hip abductors (outer thighs) and hip adductors (inner thighs). They distribute weight at the hips.

MODIFICATION

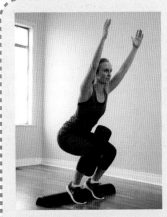

To make it easier, place a half roller beneath your heels to allow your hips to descend deeper.

HIP FLEXOR RELEASE

Hips become easily taut and sensitive when you sit often – in the car, at your desk, or on the sofa. Use this exercise to lengthen and restore flexibility to your hip flexors, which tend to be one of the most universally inhibited muscle groups.

TARGETED MUSCLES

This exercise targets the primary hip flexors, the *psoas* and *iliacus*, which originate in the pelvis and insert in the upper leg. They're responsible for moving the hips.

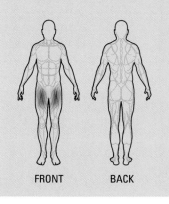

FRONT   BACK

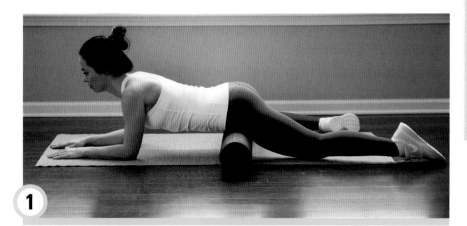

1

Lie on your stomach and place the foam roller beneath your left hip. Leave your right leg on the ground and prop yourself up onto your forearms.

HOW IT HELPS
Releasing tension in the hip flexors alleviates chronic lower back pain by restoring balance to the lower back and pelvic junction.

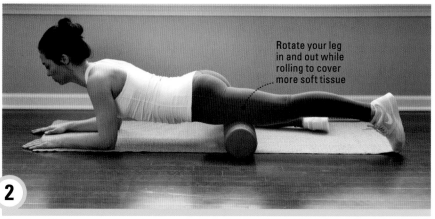

Rotate your leg in and out while rolling to cover more soft tissue

2

Slowly roll from your waistline to mid-thigh for 20 to 30 seconds, pushing and pulling with your arms and right leg. Then switch the roller to your right hip and repeat the exercise.

TARGETED HIP FLEXOR RELEASE

When your hip flexors are shortened, as they are when seated, the muscles receive poor circulation and can develop knots. Strenuous running and climbing also contributes to these painful spots. Do this release to restore health to the hip flexors.

TARGETED MUSCLES

This exercise targets the primary hip flexors, the *psoas* and *iliacus*, which originate in the pelvis and insert in the upper leg. They assist with standing and walking.

FRONT   BACK

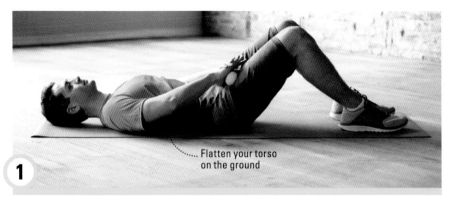

Flatten your torso on the ground

1

Lie on your back and bend your knees. Place the massage ball on your right hip flexors, halfway between your navel and right hipbone.

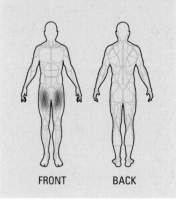

Push with your opposite hand and roll the ball in circular motions to massage your hip flexors.

2

Lower your right knee and roll the ball over your hip flexors for 20 to 30 seconds. Then lower your left knee and repeat the exercise on the left hip flexors.

TIP
If your hips are tight and inflexible, place a few pillows beneath your knee to create a comfortable lift.

TARGETED HIP ROTATOR RELEASE

The *piriformis* is a small hip rotator buried beneath the gluteal group. It's easily inflamed by extensive sitting or standing, causing the muscle to compress the sciatic nerve. Knots in this muscle are debilitating, so massaging it is vital for your health.

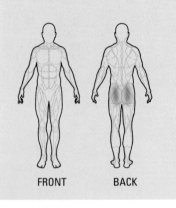
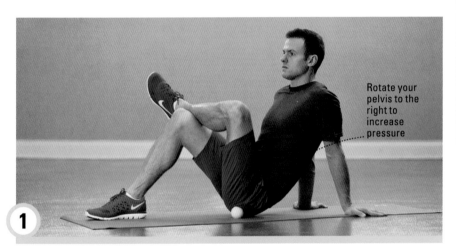

Rotate your pelvis to the right to increase pressure

1

Sit on the ground and place the massage ball beneath your left gluteals. Cross your left ankle over your right knee.

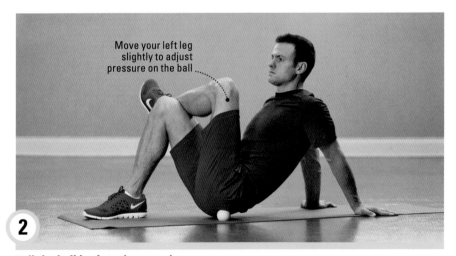

Move your left leg slightly to adjust pressure on the ball

2

Roll the ball back to the area above your gluteals, pushing with your arms.

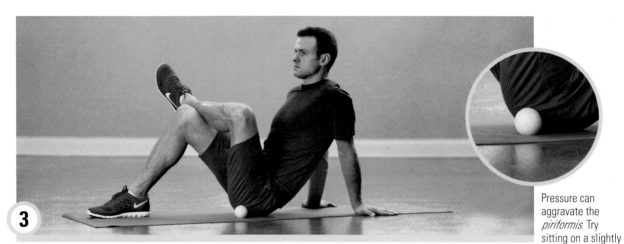

3

Roll the ball forwards to the centre of the gluteals. Continue to roll the length of the left *piriformis* for 20 to 30 seconds.

Pressure can aggravate the *piriformis*. Try sitting on a slightly cushioned surface to alleviate pain.

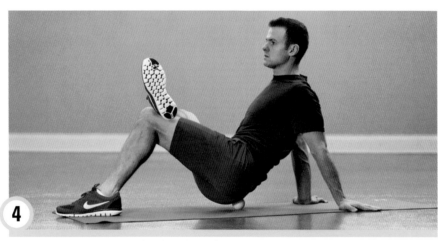

4

Switch the ball to your right gluteals and repeat the exercise.

TIP

To alleviate sciatic nerve pressure after you've released trigger points in the *piriformis*, strengthen the muscle. Try the Clamshell hip rotation.

MODIFICATION

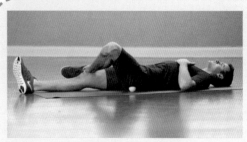

To decrease pressure, bend the targeted leg and place the ball beneath the gluteals.

HIP ROTATOR RAISE

To ensure safe lower extremity movement, this exercise activates the deeper muscles of the hip. These rotate your hips so you don't fall over when walking, but their inactivity leads to problems such as sciatica and overworked peripheral muscles.

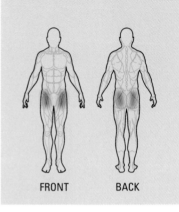

TARGETED MUSCLES

This exercise targets the *piriformis*, a deep rotator muscle of the hip that lies underneath the gluteal group. It laterally rotates and stabilizes the hip joint.

FRONT   BACK

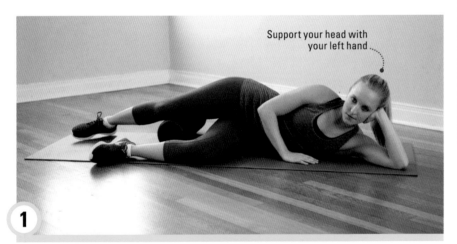

Support your head with your left hand

1

Lie on your left side, straighten your right leg, and place the foam roller beneath your right knee. Bend your left knee and hip to 90 degrees.

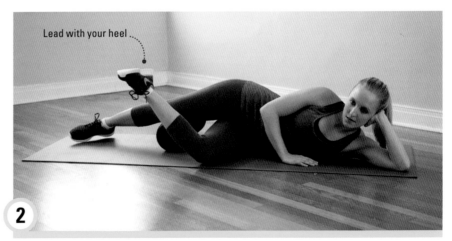

Lead with your heel

2

Anchor your left thigh and knee in position and slowly rotate your left leg up from the hip until it reaches its maximum rotation.

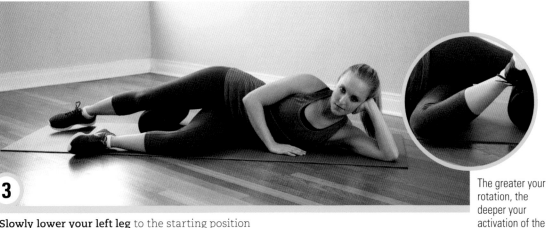

3

Slowly lower your left leg to the starting position and repeat the exercise 10 to 15 times.

The greater your rotation, the deeper your activation of the hip rotators.

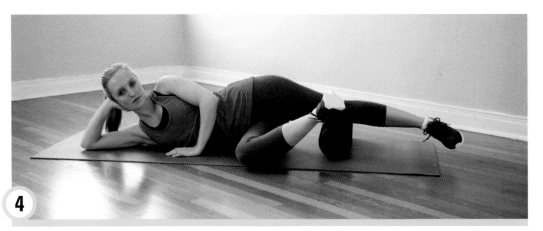

4

Roll over and repeat the exercise 10 to 15 times for your right hip rotator.

MODIFICATION

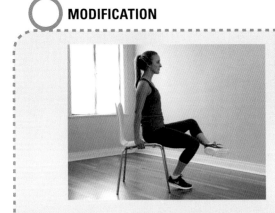

To make it easier, sit on the edge of a chair and rotate your leg in front of you to allow more latitude.

TIP

To maximize the deep contraction of the hip, relax the peripheral muscles. Contracting a small muscle like the *piriformis* is difficult if larger muscles are also active.

CLAMSHELL HIP ROTATION

This exercise strengthens the outer thighs to limit your susceptibility to injury and to combat leg ailments such as runner's knee. Activate your muscles with this rotation before a workout to keep the knee joints properly aligned with the ankles and hips.

TARGETED MUSCLES

This exercise targets the *gluteus medius* and *tensor fascia latae*, the hip abductors that originate in the pelvis and extend down the upper leg. They stabilize the knee and pelvis and pull the leg outwards.

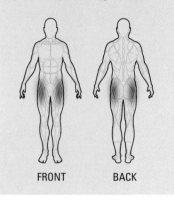

FRONT   BACK

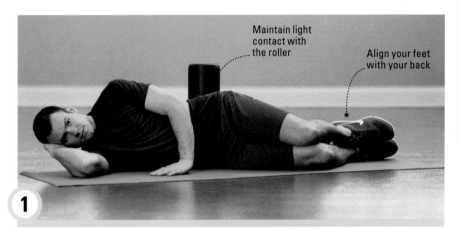

Maintain light contact with the roller

Align your feet with your back

1

Lie on your right side, stack your legs, and bend your knees to 90 degrees. Place the foam roller behind your pelvis.

HOW IT HELPS
Strengthening your gluteals ensures that your pelvis is stable when you activate the hips. This prevents injury and eases lower back pain.

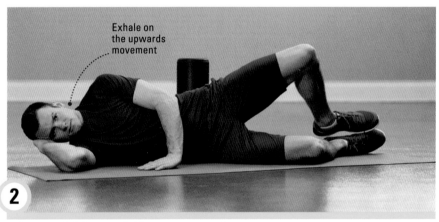

Exhale on the upwards movement

2

Raise your left knee as high as you can and hold it for 1 second. Keep your torso still.

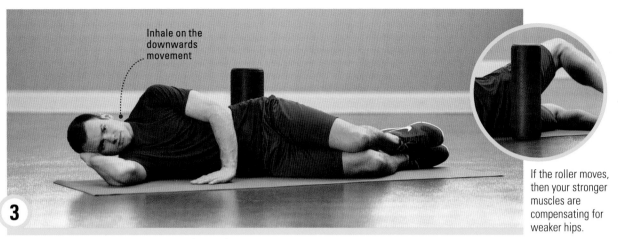

Inhale on the downwards movement

If the roller moves, then your stronger muscles are compensating for weaker hips.

3

Return your leg to the starting position and repeat the exercise 15 times with your left leg.

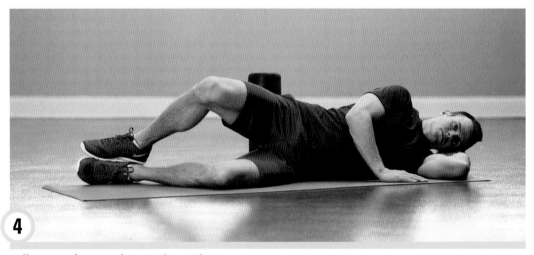

4

Roll over and repeat the exercise 15 times with your right leg.

TIP
To make it harder, ask a partner to apply pressure with his or her hands to the outside of your moving knee during the movement.

GLUTEAL GROUP RELEASE

If you spend a lot of time sitting down, your gluteals – the muscles that keep you upright from the hips – are likely to be underused. Rolling this area restores hip flexibility to stabilize your lower back and knees. It's a great addition to a warm-up routine before working out.

TARGETED MUSCLES

This exercise targets the *gluteus maximus*, *medius*, and *minimus*, which are located at the backside of the pelvis. The gluteal muscles keep the body upright.

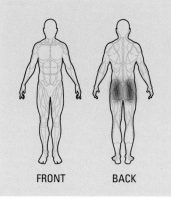

FRONT   BACK

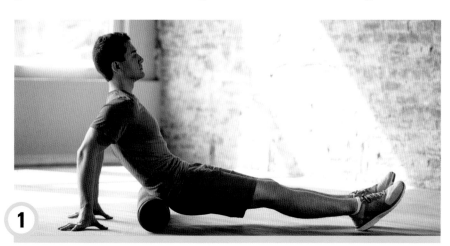

1

Sit on the foam roller and place both hands on the ground behind you to hold yourself upright. Extend your legs.

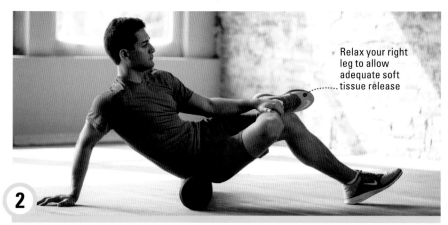

Relax your right leg to allow adequate soft tissue release

2

Rest your right ankle on your left knee and shift your weight to the gluteals of the right leg. Bend your left knee to increase pressure.

HOW IT HELPS

This exercise relieves pain from sciatica, a disorder caused by excessive pressure on the sciatic nerve, which runs beneath the gluteal group.

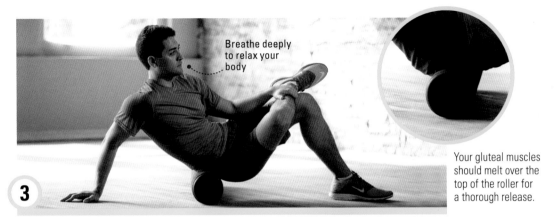

Breathe deeply
to relax your
body

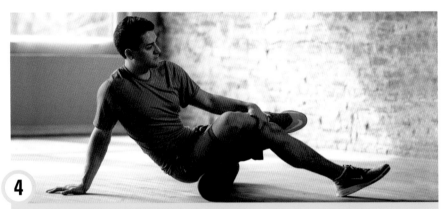

Your gluteal muscles
should melt over the
top of the roller for
a thorough release.

3 **Roll back** to your waistline,
pushing with your right arm
and pulling with your left foot.

4 **Roll forwards** to the top of your thigh. Continue
to roll back and forth over the length of the right
gluteals for 20 to 30 seconds.

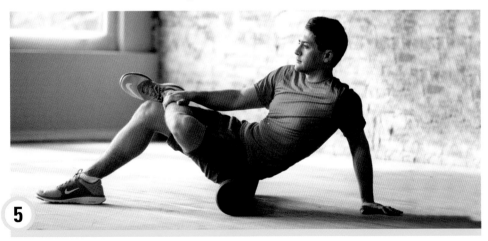

5 **Uncross your legs and repeat** the exercise
for your left gluteals.

TARGETED GLUTEAL GROUP RELEASE

Many movements (or a lack of movement) can cause knots to develop throughout your gluteal group. While foam rolling the gluteals restores flexibility, using a massage ball to address the knots makes the muscles more healthy and pain-free.

TARGETED MUSCLES

This exercises targets the *gluteus maximus* and *gluteus medius*. They keep the body upright from the hip and help stabilize the pelvis.

FRONT   BACK

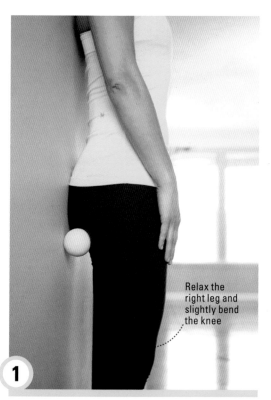

Relax the right leg and slightly bend the knee

1

Stand upright and pin the ball between the wall and the thickest point of your right gluteals. Lean into the ball.

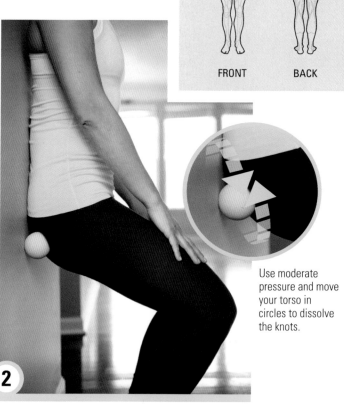

Use moderate pressure and move your torso in circles to dissolve the knots.

2

Bend your knees to roll the ball over the gluteals. If you find a painful point, massage it with circular movements for 20 to 30 seconds.

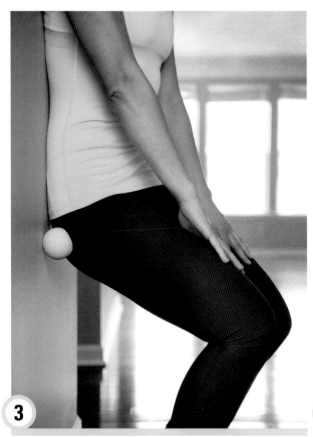

3

Rotate your pelvis to the right and refocus pressure on your outer right gluteals. Roll your muscles over the ball, and spend 20 to 30 seconds massaging particularly painful points.

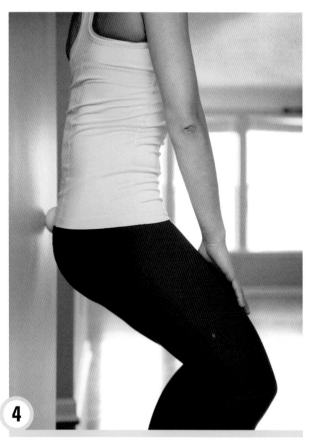

4

Switch the ball to your left gluteals and repeat the exercise.

TIP

To avoid underworking the *gluteus medius*, break up long periods of sitting with small walks. Sitting restricts circulation to the gluteals and causes knots to develop.

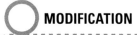

MODIFICATION

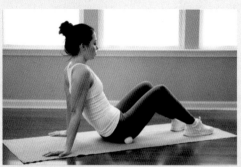

To increase pressure, sit on the ground and place the ball beneath your gluteals.

GLUTEAL BRIDGE

Because the gluteals are commonly underused, the Gluteal bridge strengthens the muscles and restores balance to surrounding tissue. If you sit in your car or at your desk a lot, the exercise can significantly improve your quality of movement.

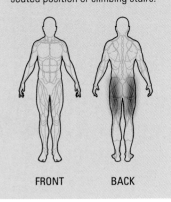
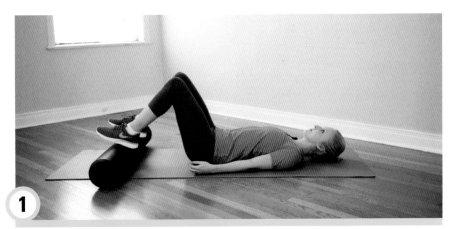

1

Lie on your back and lay your arms at your sides. Put your feet hip-width apart on the foam roller and bend your knees to 90 degrees.

CAUTION
To avoid straining your lower back, create outward pressure in your lower abdomen and maintain the slight, neutral curves in your spine.

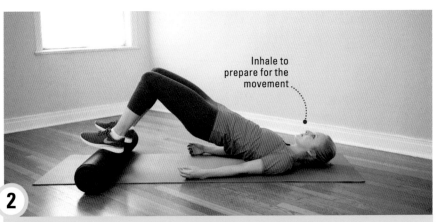

Inhale to prepare for the movement

2

Raise your hips until they're aligned with your thighs and you feel your gluteals contract.

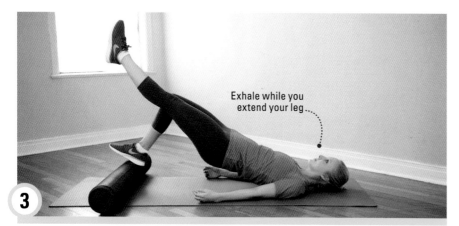

Exhale while you
extend your leg...

3

Keep your hips raised and
extend your left leg out in
a straight line.

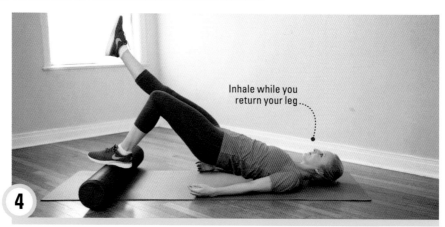

Inhale while you
return your leg...

4

Return your left leg to the foam roller and
extend your right leg, keeping your hips raised.

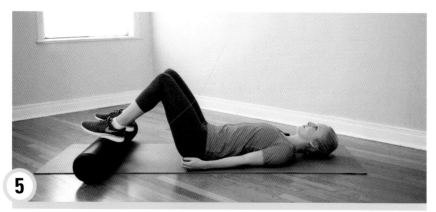

5

Return your right leg to the roller and lower your
hips to the starting position. Repeat the exercise
10 to 15 times, or until your muscles fatigue.

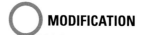 **MODIFICATION**

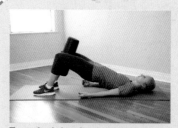

To make it harder, hold the roller
between your knees and squeeze
your inner thigh muscles.

STRAIGHT-LEG GLUTEAL BRIDGE

Sometimes hip stability and leg mobility are weak and asymmetrical. To make activities such as running more efficient, this exercise strengthens your hips, core, and hamstrings to prepare you for single-leg stances and lateral movements.

TARGETED MUSCLES

This exercise targets the gluteal group, hamstrings, and abdomen. They stabilize the pelvis and enable hip mobility.

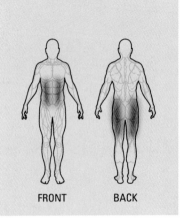

FRONT   BACK

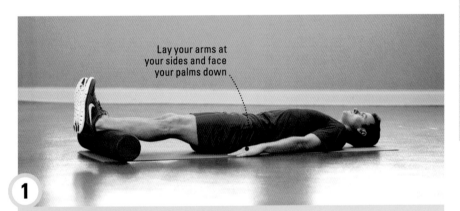

Lay your arms at your sides and face your palms down

1

Lie on your back and place the foam roller beneath your ankles. Straighten your legs and point your toes upwards.

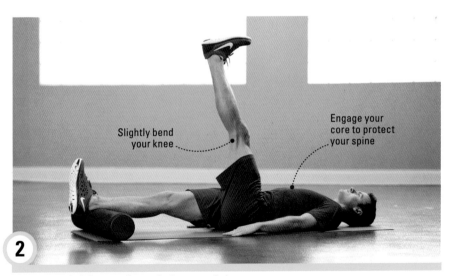

Slightly bend your knee

Engage your core to protect your spine

CAUTION
To avoid straining your lower back, do not use it to propel the exercise. As a preventative measure, push your lower back into the ground.

2

Raise your left leg until you feel a stretch in the back of your left hamstrings.

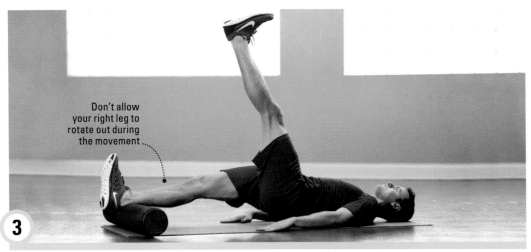

Don't allow your right leg to rotate out during the movement

3

Contract your right gluteals and lift your hips 8–15cm (3–6in) off the ground.

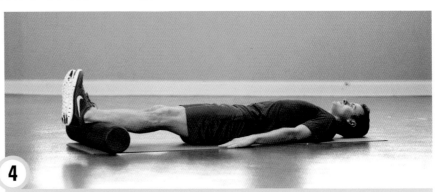

4

After 2 seconds, lower your hips and leg. Repeat the exercise 10 times with your left leg.

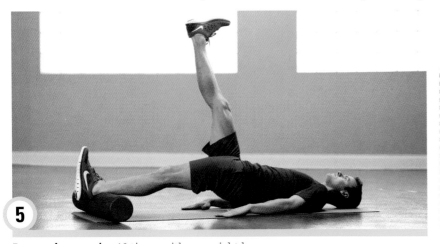

5

Repeat the exercise 10 times with your right leg.

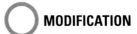

MODIFICATION

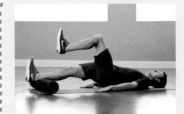

To make it easier, bend your knee to 90 degrees if the hamstrings of your raised leg are too tight.

QUADRICEPS RELEASE

Rolling your quadriceps is a quick way to improve knee and lower back health. Flexible knee joints allow the hamstrings to fully contract, which in turn balances tension in surrounding areas. This release is great after a long day of driving or sitting.

TARGETED MUSCLES

This exercise targets the four muscles that compose the quadriceps, which originate at the hip and end at the knee. They extend the knee and flex the hip.

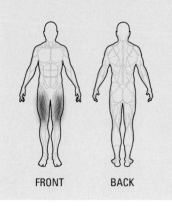

FRONT   BACK

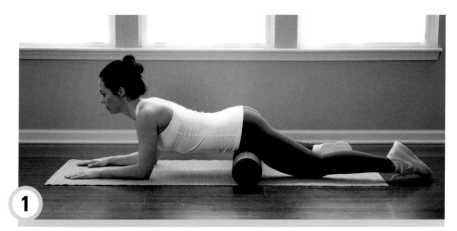

1

Lie on your stomach and place the foam roller beneath your left thigh. Leave your right leg on the ground and prop yourself up on your forearms.

HOW IT HELPS
Massaging the quadriceps balances overworked muscles in the entire leg. It loosens the knee joint, allowing full hamstring contraction.

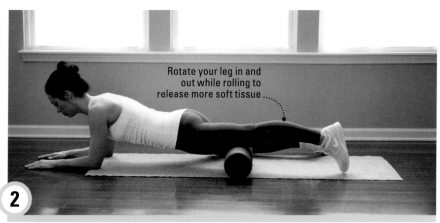

Rotate your leg in and out while rolling to release more soft tissue

2

Roll down to your knee, pulling with your arms and your right leg.

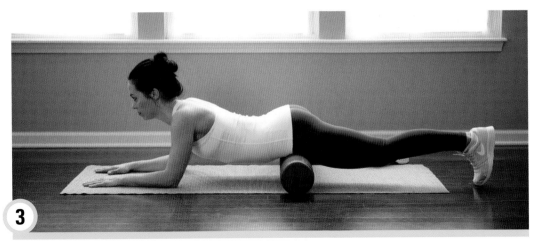

3

Roll up to the top of your thigh. Continue to roll the length of the quadriceps for 30 to 40 seconds.

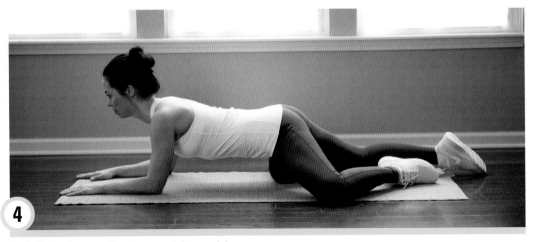

4

Switch the foam roller to your right quadriceps and repeat the exercise.

MODIFICATIONS

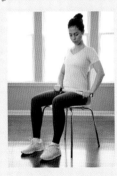

To make it easier, sit on a chair and use a massage stick to roll your quadriceps.

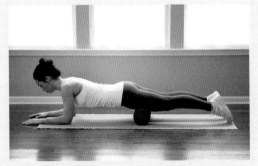

To decrease pressure, place both legs side by side on the roller.

TARGETED QUADRICEPS RELEASE

The quadriceps muscle group is large and powerful, and knots that form here can lead to pain around the knee and hips. It's great to do this exercise frequently because releasing the quadriceps can significantly alleviate pain in your lower body.

TARGETED MUSCLES

This exercise targets the four heads of the quadriceps muscle group in the front thigh: the *rectus femoris*, *vastus lateralis*, *vastus intermedius*, and *vastus medialis*. They contribute to knee extension.

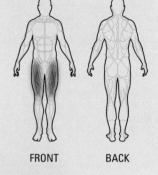

FRONT   BACK

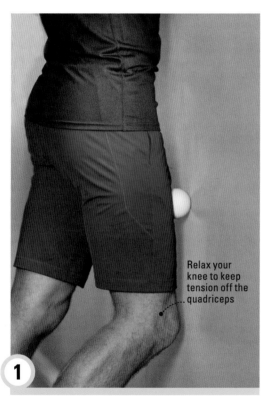

Relax your knee to keep tension off the quadriceps

1 **Slightly bend your right knee** and pin the lacrosse ball between the wall and the middle of your right quadriceps. Lean into the ball.

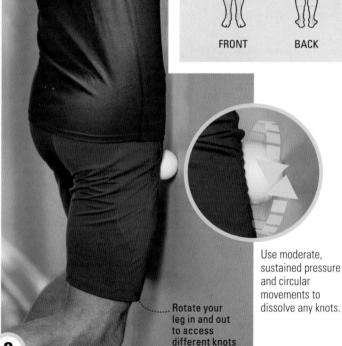

Rotate your leg in and out to access different knots

Use moderate, sustained pressure and circular movements to dissolve any knots.

2 **Bend your knees** to roll the ball up to your hip. If you find a painful point, massage it with circular movements for 20 to 30 seconds.

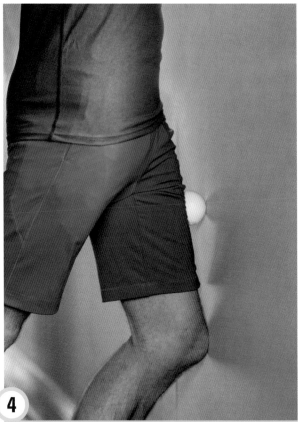

4

Switch the lacrosse ball to your left leg and repeat the exercise for your left quadriceps.

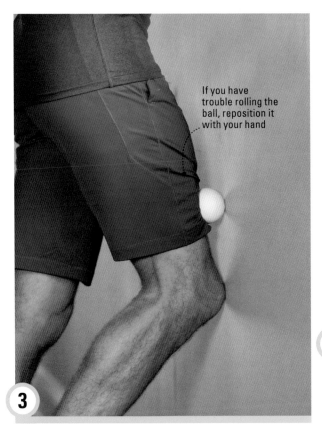

If you have trouble rolling the ball, reposition it with your hand

3

Straighten your knees to allow the ball to roll down to your knee, and spend 20 to 30 seconds massaging any particularly painful points.

HOW IT HELPS

Because the *rectus femoris* contributes to bending the hip, this exercise helps people who sit all day and have referred pain and knots.

MODIFICATION

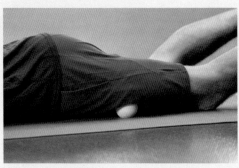

To increase pressure, lie on the ground and place the lacrosse ball beneath the quadriceps.

OUTER THIGH AND HIP RELEASE

This is one of the most popular foam rolling exercises because it releases the often overworked outer thigh. The massage targets the primary lateral stabilizers of the knee joint, which can be tight because of inactive hip and thigh adductors.

TARGETED MUSCLES

This exercise targets the *tensor fascia latae* (TFL) muscle, which is linked to the *iliotibial* (IT) band, a ligament that runs down the outside of the thigh. They stabilize the pelvis and the knee.

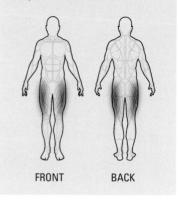

FRONT   BACK

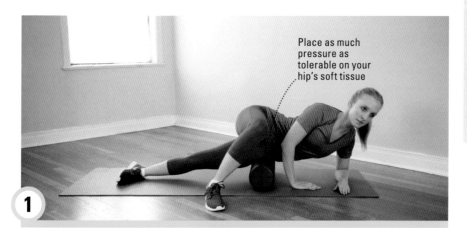

Place as much pressure as tolerable on your hip's soft tissue

1

Lie on your left side and place the foam roller beneath your left hip. Plant your right foot on the ground and prop yourself up on your left forearm.

TIP
To make the exercise easier and more comfortable, sit in a chair, rest your feet on the ground, and roll the area with a massage stick.

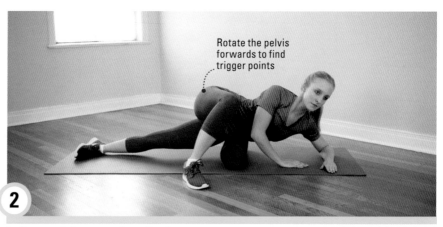

Rotate the pelvis forwards to find trigger points

2

Roll up and down on the roller for 20 to 30 seconds between the bony parts of your hip and pelvis bones. Then switch the roller to your right hip and repeat the exercise.

TARGETED OUTER HIP RELEASE

This targeted trigger point exercise directly releases points of tenderness in the hip, especially for athletes. Alleviating this area lengthens the IT band, which runs down the outside of your upper leg. Perform this release to improve total leg circulation.

TARGETED MUSCLES

This exercise targets the *tensor fascia latae* (TFL), an outer hip muscle, and the *gluteus medius*, an outer buttocks muscle. They stabilize lateral knee movement.

FRONT   BACK

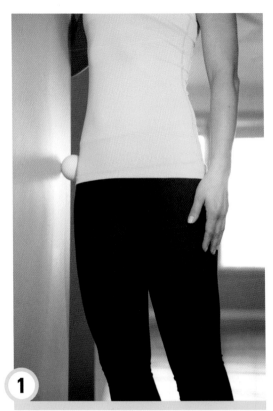

1 **Stand upright** and pin the massage ball between the wall and the soft tissues of your right hip. Lean into the ball.

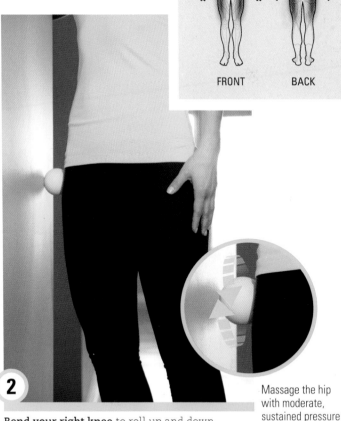

2 **Bend your right knee** to roll up and down over the hip for 20 to 30 seconds. Then repeat the exercise on your left hip.

Massage the hip with moderate, sustained pressure and circular movements until pain dissipates.

HAMSTRINGS RELEASE

Muscles are most efficient when you use them at many lengths, so if you're sitting or standing all day with inactive knees and hips, your hamstrings are most likely to be tight. Rolling out this tension relieves referred lower back and knee pain.

TARGETED MUSCLES

This exercise targets the three muscles that compose the hamstrings, located at the back of the thigh. They bend the knee and extend the hip.

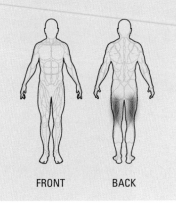

FRONT   BACK

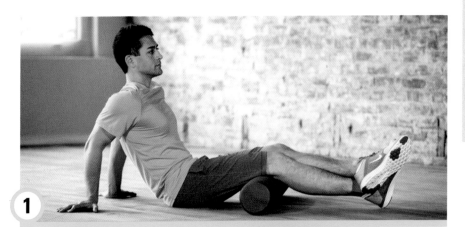

1

Sit on the ground and place the foam roller beneath your right hamstrings. Cross your left ankle over your right ankle.

TIP
So that your hamstrings are receptive to self-myofascial release, relax your feet and maintain deep, conscious breathing.

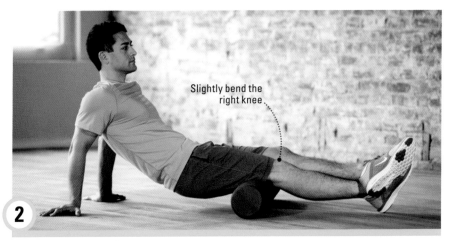

Slightly bend the right knee

2

Lift your hips and roll up to your rear, pushing with your arms.

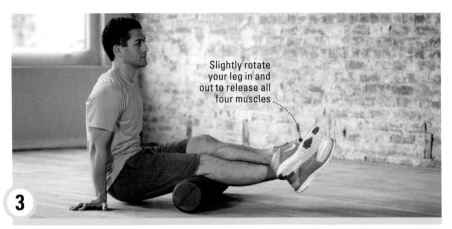

Slightly rotate
your leg in and
out to release all
four muscles

3

Roll down to your right knee. Continue rolling
the length of the hamstrings for 30 to 40 seconds.

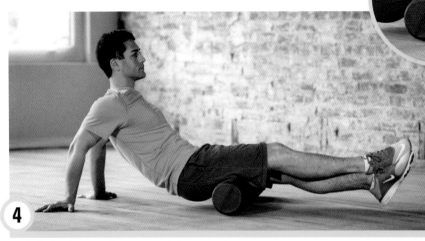

The hamstrings
require immense
pressure to
release, so push
your weight down
into the roller.

4

Switch the foam roller to your left hamstrings
and repeat the exercise.

MODIFICATIONS

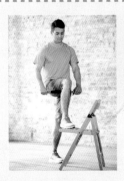

**To make it
easier,** place
your foot on a
chair and use a
massage stick
to roll your
hamstrings.

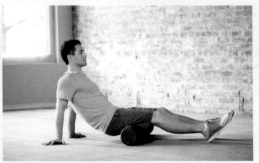

**To decrease
pressure,**
uncross your
ankles and roll
both legs at the
same time.

TARGETED HAMSTRINGS RELEASE

Releasing hamstring trigger points starts a beneficial chain reaction that improves total body health. This exercise alleviates pain in the knee and in the back of the thigh. It can even heal headaches and referred pain in your neck caused by short, taut hamstrings.

TARGETED MUSCLES

This exercise targets the three muscles of the hamstrings: the *biceps femoris, semitendinosus,* and *semimembranosus.* They create hip flexion and extension.

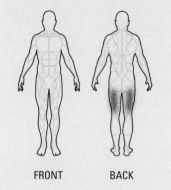

FRONT   BACK

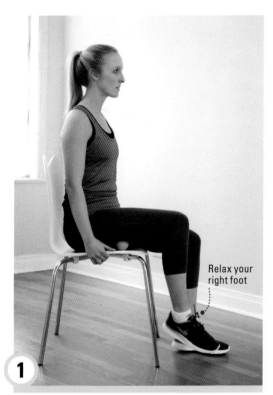

Relax your right foot

1

Sit on a chair and place the massage ball beneath your right thigh. Bend your right knee to 90 degrees and hold the sides of the chair.

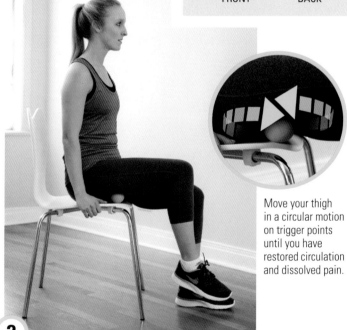

Move your thigh in a circular motion on trigger points until you have restored circulation and dissolved pain.

2

Roll the ball back to your rear by sliding forwards. If you find a painful point, massage it with circular movements for 20 to 30 seconds.

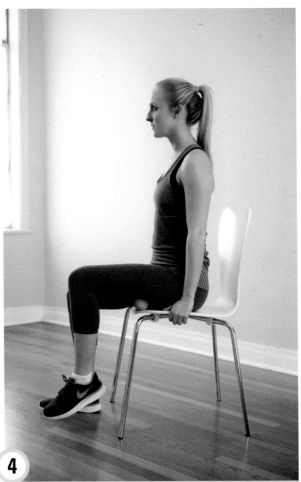

4

Switch the ball to your left thigh and repeat the exercise for your left hamstrings.

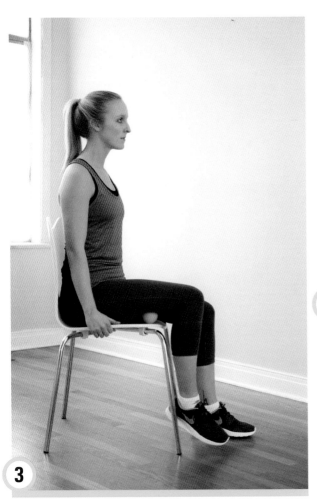

3

Roll the ball forwards to your knee by sliding back in the chair, and spend 20 to 30 seconds massaging any particularly painful points.

TIP

To increase pressure on a trigger point, grasp the sides of the chair and pull yourself into the ball. Moderate pressure is best to dissolve these painful spots.

INNER THIGH RELEASE

This exercise activates the deep muscles of the hip to ensure safe lower extremity movement. Your inner thighs rotate the hips so you stay erect when walking, but their inactivity leads to problems such as sciatica and other overworked muscles.

TARGETED MUSCLES

This exercise targets the adductor muscle group, which runs from the top of the inner thigh to the inside of the knee. These muscles laterally stabilize the knee joint and help to stabilize the pelvis.

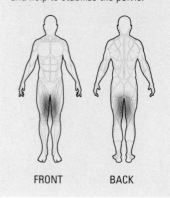

FRONT   BACK

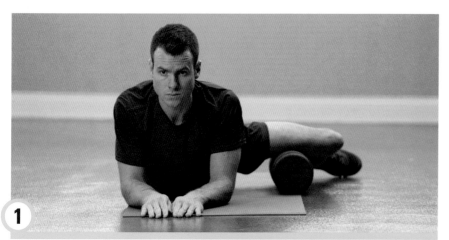

1

Lie on your stomach, prop yourself up on your forearms, and bend your left hip and knee to 90 degrees. Place the foam roller beneath your left thigh.

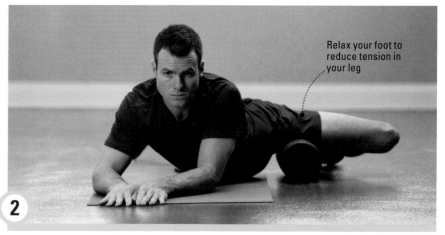

Relax your foot to reduce tension in your leg

2

Roll up to your groin, pushing yourself to the left with your arms and right leg.

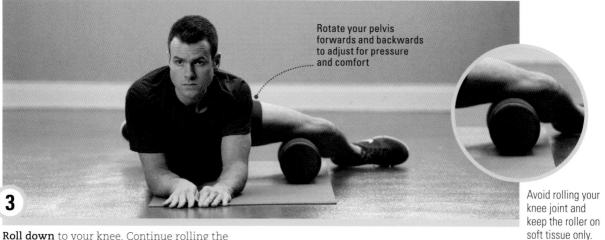

Rotate your pelvis forwards and backwards to adjust for pressure and comfort

Avoid rolling your knee joint and keep the roller on soft tissue only.

3

Roll down to your knee. Continue rolling the length of the inner thigh for 20 to 30 seconds.

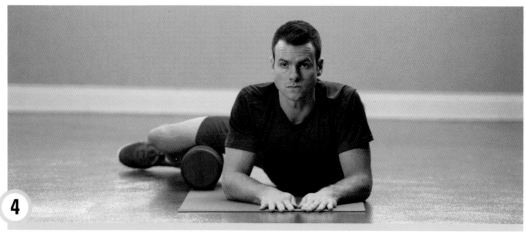

4

Switch the foam roller to your right inner thigh and repeat the exercise.

MODIFICATION

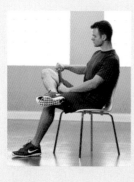

To make it easier, sit on a chair, cross your ankle over your knee to access the inner thigh, and use a massage stick to roll the muscles.

HOW IT HELPS

Rolling the inner thigh reduces tightness in the outer thigh. Self-myofascial release balances muscle groups that pull on each other.

TARGETED INNER THIGH RELEASE

Single leg-stance movements such as walking, running, skating, and skiing demand a lot of the inner thighs. The inhibited muscles are often left untreated for knots, but massaging them is important for releasing tension in the overused area.

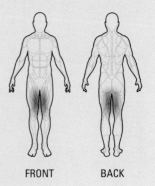

TARGETED MUSCLES

This exercise targets the *adductor longus, adductor brevis*, and *adductor magnus*, the inner thigh hip muscles. They pull the legs towards the body's midline.

FRONT   BACK

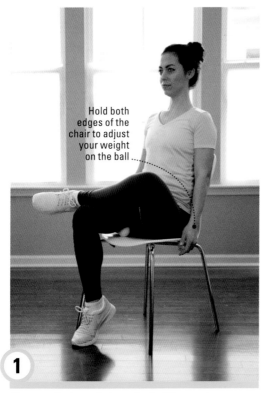

Hold both edges of the chair to adjust your weight on the ball ...

1

Sit on a chair and place the ball beneath your right inner thigh. Cross your left ankle over your knee and maintain weight on your right leg.

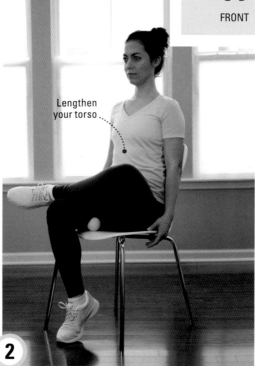

Lengthen your torso ...

2

Roll the ball forwards to your knee by sliding backwards. If you find a painful point, massage it with circular movements for about 25 seconds.

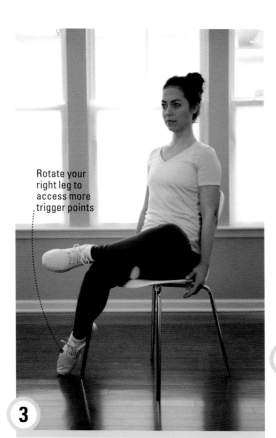

Rotate your right leg to access more trigger points

3

Roll the ball back to your rear by sliding forwards. Spend 20 to 30 seconds massaging any painful points.

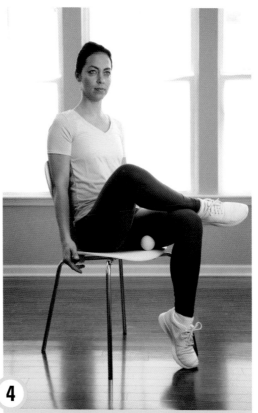

4

Switch the ball to your left inner thigh and repeat the exercise.

HOW IT HELPS
This exercise releases knots caused by a heavy fall. Your inner thighs rapidly activate to stop a fall, but a fast reaction can strain the muscles.

MODIFICATION

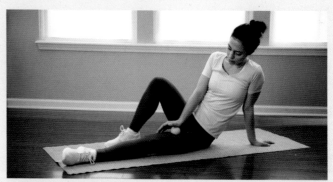

To decrease pressure, use your opposite hand to press the ball into your inner thigh.

KNEE RELEASE

The small movement of this exercise releases tension in the knee joint, which becomes strained when you sit or stand all day. It's especially beneficial before any lower body workouts so that your leg muscles are flexible and less prone to injuries.

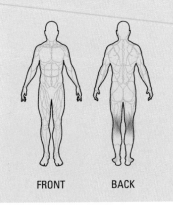
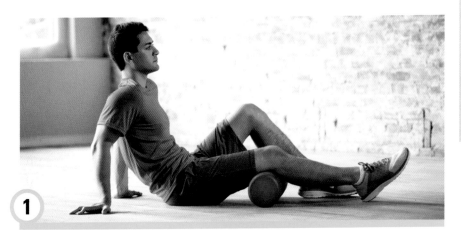

(1)

Sit on the ground, place the foam roller beneath your right knee, and plant your left foot on the ground for support.

HOW IT HELPS
Releasing the knee joint helps the major leg muscles function properly. The *popliteus* assists several muscles during exercise, but it's easily overworked.

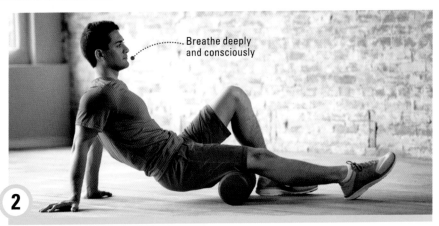

Breathe deeply and consciously

(2)

Lift your hips and slightly bend your right knee. Roll up to your thigh, pushing with your arms and pulling with your left foot.

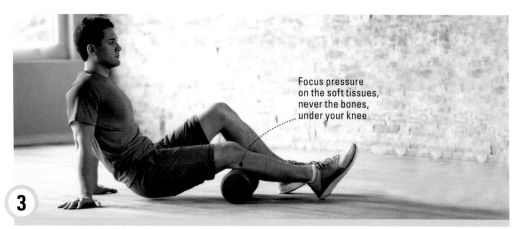

Focus pressure
on the soft tissues,
never the bones,
under your knee

3

Roll down to the top of your calf. Continue rolling
the length of your knee for 20 to 30 seconds.

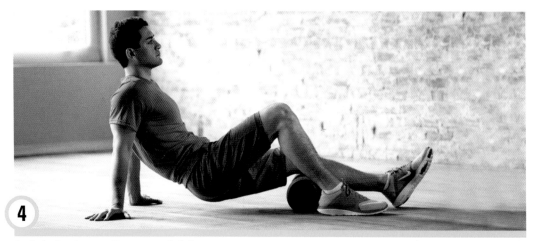

4

Switch the foam roller to your left knee
and repeat the exercise.

MODIFICATIONS

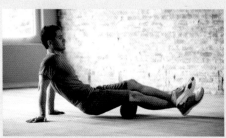

To increase pressure, cross your ankles and shift
your weight to the targeted soft tissues.

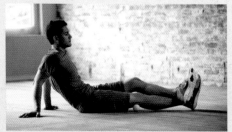

For more targeted pressure, use a ball to
pinpoint the small muscle.

SHIN RELEASE

Easily overused by repetitive movement on hard surfaces, the muscles around your shin bone can become tense and painful. Massage the shin muscles before lower body impact activities to improve the way your legs absorb the vibrations.

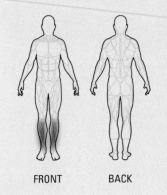

TARGETED MUSCLES

This exercise targets the *tibialis anterior* and the *extensor digitorum longus* muscles, both located next to the tibia (shin bone). They control several foot movements.

FRONT   BACK

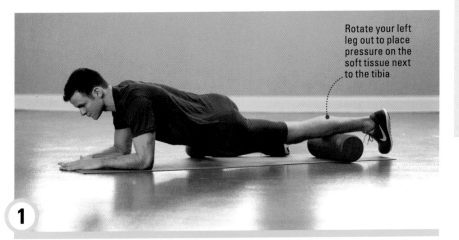

Rotate your left leg out to place pressure on the soft tissue next to the tibia

1

Lie on your stomach, place the foam roller beneath your left shin, and put your right knee out to the side for leverage. Prop yourself up on your forearms.

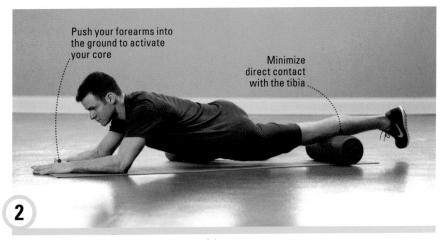

Push your forearms into the ground to activate your core

Minimize direct contact with the tibia

2

Roll up to the bottom of your knee, pushing with your arms and your right knee.

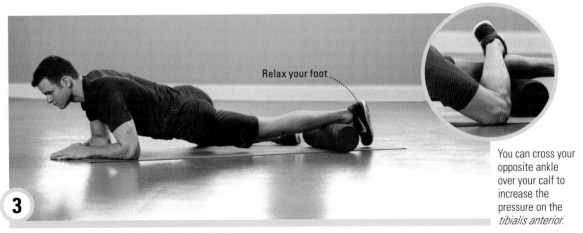

Relax your foot

You can cross your opposite ankle over your calf to increase the pressure on the *tibialis anterior*.

3

Roll down to your ankle. Continue to roll the length of your shin for 20 to 30 seconds.

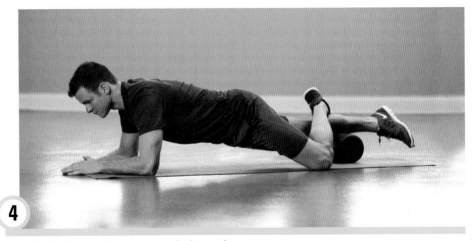

4

Switch the foam roller to your right leg and repeat the exercise.

TIP
To ease pain from shin splints, release the *tibialis anterior* frequently. Runners and cyclists are often victims of this inflamed muscle, which exacerbates the pain.

MODIFICATION

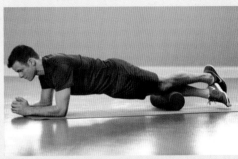

To increase pressure, cross your feet and focus your weight onto one leg.

TARGETED SHIN RELEASE

If you're frequently moving around on uneven surfaces, the front of your lower legs may become laden with knots, which refer pain to your feet. Perform this exercise to release the pain and tension around the shins, big toes, and calves.

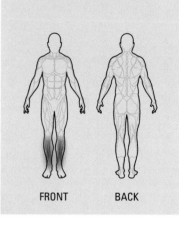

TARGETED MUSCLES

This exercise targets the *tibialis anterior*, located at the outer side of the tibia (shin bone). It controls several movements of the foot.

FRONT   BACK

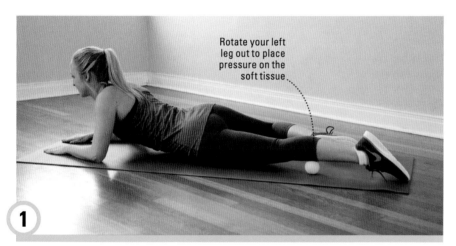

Rotate your left leg out to place pressure on the soft tissue

1

Lie on your stomach and place the ball beneath your left shin. Put your right knee out to the side for leverage.

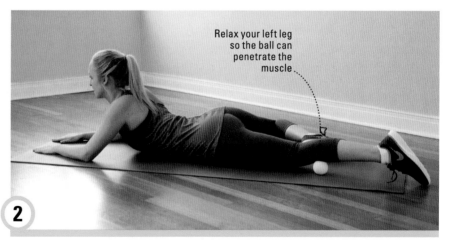

Relax your left leg so the ball can penetrate the muscle

2

Roll the ball up to your knee, pushing with your arms and your right knee. If you find a particularly painful point, massage it with circular movements for 20 to 30 seconds.

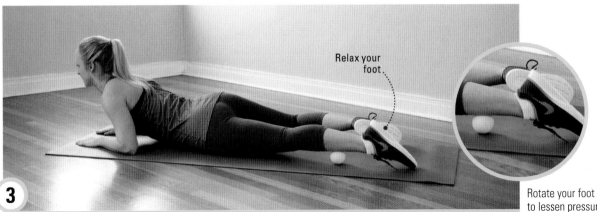

Relax your foot

3

Roll the ball down to the ankle, and spend 20 to 30 seconds massaging painful points.

Rotate your foot to lessen pressure on the shin bone, and use sustained, circular motions to treat the knots.

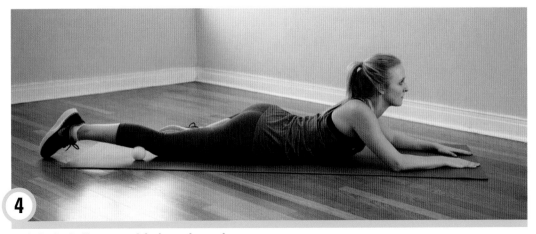

4

Switch the ball to your right lower leg and repeat the exercise.

CAUTION
To avoid irritating already inflamed soft tissue, don't place too much pressure too soon on the muscle. Gradually increase the pressure each time.

MODIFICATION

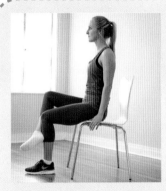

To make it easier, sit on a chair and use your heel to penetrate any knots.

CALF MASSAGE

With many occupational hazards, the calf muscles can become overused, tight, and unresponsive, but this exercise restores them to proper function. Roll the area before lower body workouts, especially ballistic exercises that involve jumping.

TARGETED MUSCLES

This exercise targets the *tibialis posterior, gastrocnemius,* and *soleus,* the calf muscles. They control movements of the foot such as pointing the toes.

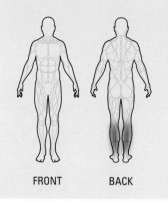

FRONT   BACK

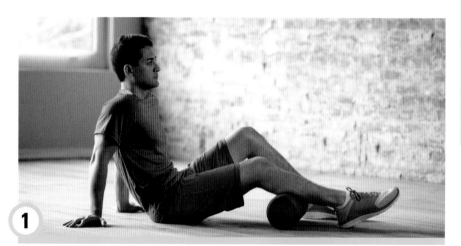

1

Sit on the ground, place the foam roller beneath your right calf, and plant your left foot on the ground for support.

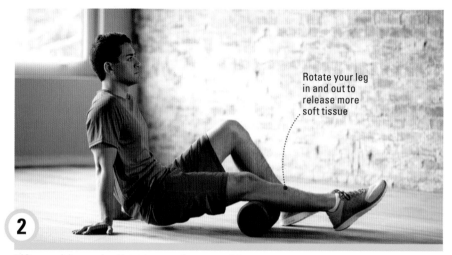

Rotate your leg in and out to release more soft tissue

2

Lift your hips and roll up to your knee, pushing with your arms and left foot.

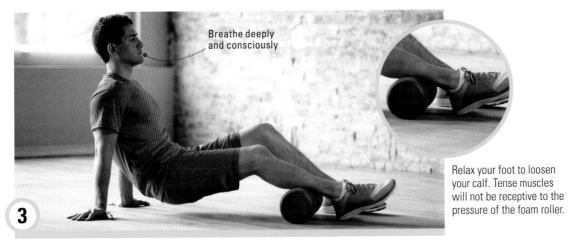

Breathe deeply
and consciously

Relax your foot to loosen
your calf. Tense muscles
will not be receptive to the
pressure of the foam roller.

3

Roll down to your ankle. Continue rolling up and
down the length of the calf for 20 to 30 seconds.

HOW IT HELPS
Massaging the calves
improves their ability
to absorb impact
and dampen vibrations.
This reduces the
chance of shin splints.

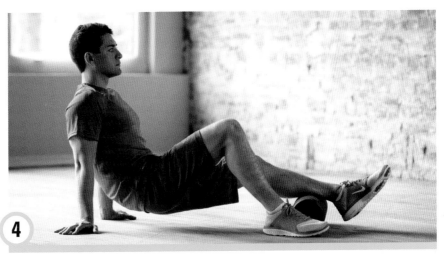

4

Switch the foam roller to your left calf and
repeat the exercise.

MODIFICATIONS

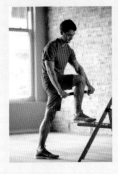

**To make it
easier,** place
your foot on a
chair and use a
massage stick.

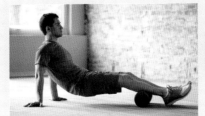

To decrease pressure, place both legs
side by side on the roller.

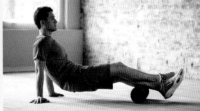

To increase pressure, cross your legs and
shift your weight onto the targeted calf.

TARGETED CALF RELEASE

This more targeted method releases knots in your calves. If you spend all day on your feet, you're a likely victim of these painful spots, but concentrating the pressure can relieve discomfort. It also helps to reduce referred pain in the ankles and feet.

TARGETED MUSCLES

This exercise targets the *gastrocnemius* and the *soleus* muscles in the calf. They're the primary flexors of the ankle.

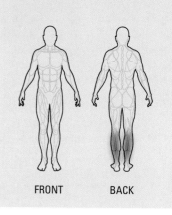

FRONT   BACK

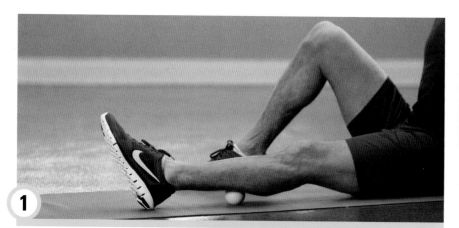

1

Sit on the ground and place the ball beneath your left calf. Plant your right foot on the ground for support.

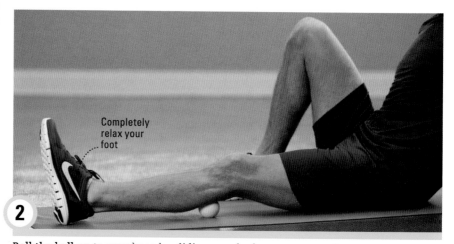

Completely relax your foot

2

Roll the ball up to your knee by sliding your body forwards. If you find a painful point, massage it with circular movements for 20 to 30 seconds.

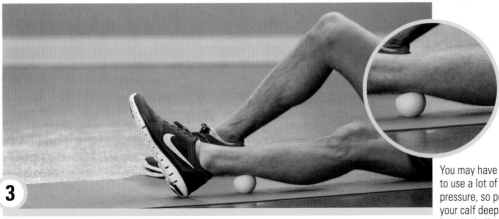

3

Roll the ball down to your ankle, and spend 20 to 30 seconds massaging any painful points.

You may have to use a lot of pressure, so push your calf deeply into the ball to restore blood flow.

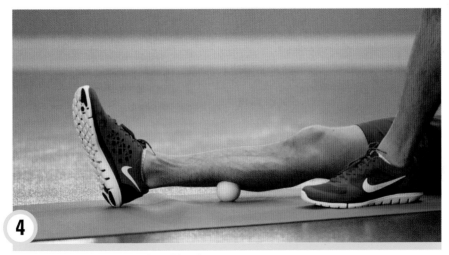

4

Switch the ball to your right calf and repeat the exercise.

HOW IT HELPS
Massaging the calves can relieve cramps. Knots do not always actively produce pain, but they can nevertheless cause sporadic spasms.

MODIFICATION

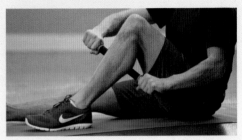

To make it easier, use a massage stick and roll the tool against the knots in your calves.

SPIRAL CALF RAISE

When walking, for example, your feet roll in and out as your hips rotate internally and externally. The Spiral calf raise develops this relationship so that your gait is more proficient, making you less prone to injury during activities that require a spiral movement.

TARGETED MUSCLES

This exercise targets the *posterior* and *anterior tibialis* (located deep within the lower leg), and the external hip rotators. They control the legs while walking.

FRONT   BACK

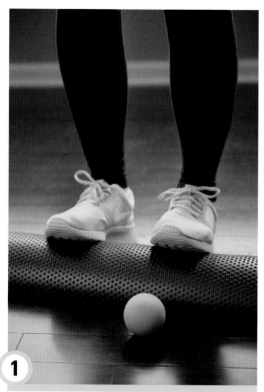

1

Stand with the balls of your feet 5–10cm (2–4in) apart on a half foam roller.

2

Squeeze the ball between your heels, just beneath the bones of your ankle joints.

Squeezing the ball teaches your ankles to align properly under your hips while walking, rather than to roll to the outside of the feet.

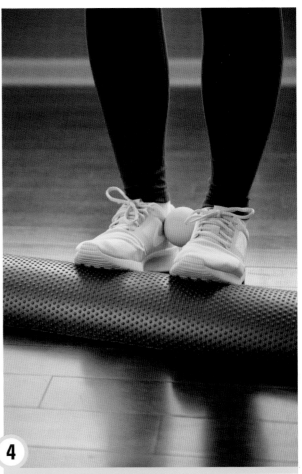

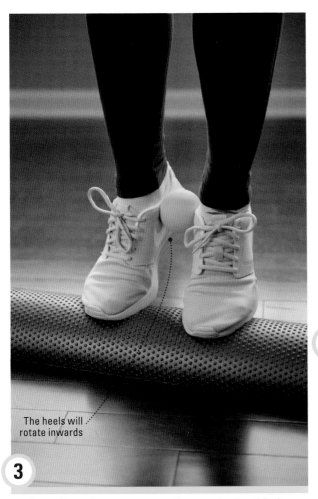

The heels will
rotate inwards

3

Push up through your toes to raise your body with the
calf muscles. Simultaneously squeeze your gluteals to
rotate your legs externally.

4

After fully contracting your calves, relax your gluteals
and slowly descend back to the starting position. Repeat
the exercise 15 times.

TIP
If it's difficult to
keep your balance,
lightly rest your hands
against a wall or on a
chair for support, or
remove your shoes.
Centre your weight
over your feet.

ANKLE RELEASE

Use this exercise to relieve tension in your primary ankle-stabilizing muscles, the peroneals. They're often overworked if you walk or run on challenging surfaces such as trails and sand, so roll them before your workout to achieve optimal movement.

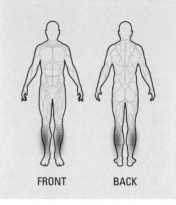

TARGETED MUSCLES

This exercise targets the *peroneus longus, brevis,* and *tertius* (the peroneals) located in the outer side of the lower leg. They control several movements of the foot.

FRONT   BACK

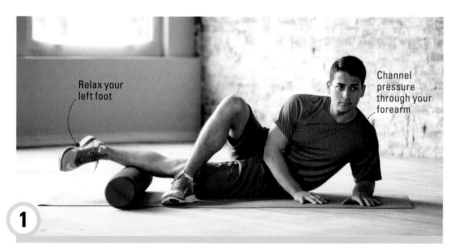

Relax your left foot

Channel pressure through your forearm

1

Lie on your left side and place the foam roller beneath your lower left leg. Plant your right foot on the ground and prop yourself up on your forearm.

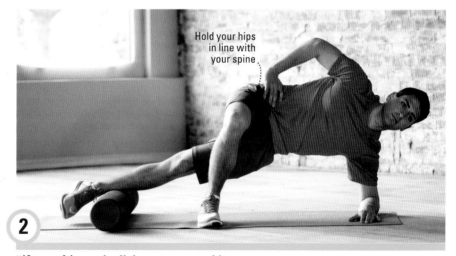

Hold your hips in line with your spine

2

Lift your hips and roll down to your ankle, pushing with your right leg.

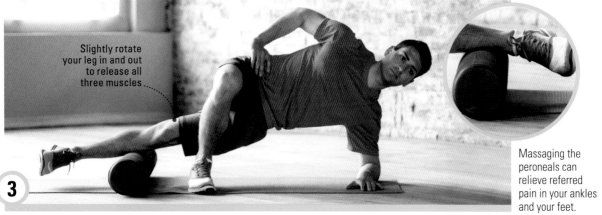

Slightly rotate your leg in and out to release all three muscles

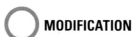

Massaging the peroneals can relieve referred pain in your ankles and your feet.

3

Roll up to your knee joint. Continue to roll the length of the lower leg for 20 to 30 seconds.

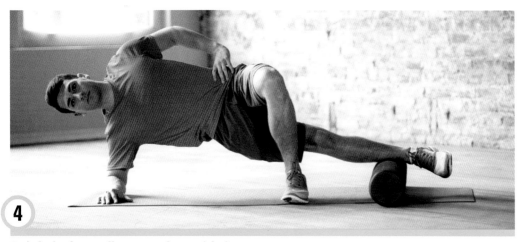

4

Switch the foam roller to your lower right leg and repeat the exercise.

CAUTION

To avoid injury, if you feel excessive pain, offset pressure from the roller. Shift your weight to your support leg and arm, and never exceed your pain tolerance.

MODIFICATION

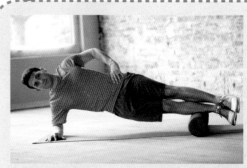

To increase pressure, stack both legs on top of the foam roller.

ARCH RELEASE

This vital exercise alleviates pain from *plantar fasciitis* and restores circulation and flexibility for healthy feet. The sole of the foot is the brain's principal input for balance and reaction time, and this exercise improves the foot's receptivity to these signals.

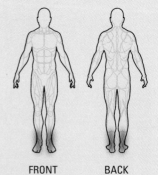
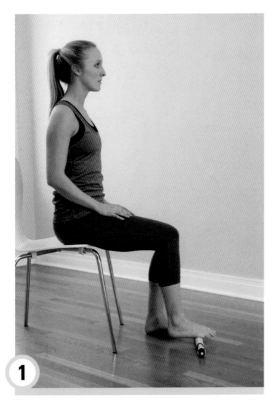

1

Sit on a chair and place the massage stick on the ground beneath your right foot.

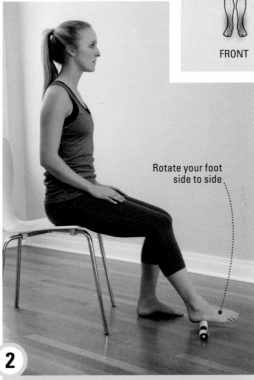

Rotate your foot side to side

2

Slide your right foot forwards and backwards over the stick, from the ball to the heel of the foot, for 30 to 45 seconds. Repeat for the left foot.

TARGETED FOOT RELEASE

A good foot massage is relaxing and restorative, but the Targeted foot release can also do wonders for relieving pain caused by knots. If you're on your feet a lot and have tight calves or wear shoes that don't fit well, this exercise will help you.

TARGETED MUSCLES

This release targets the seven primary muscles in the sole of the foot, which collectively control the toes and stabilize the arch.

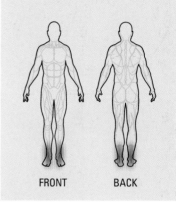

FRONT   BACK

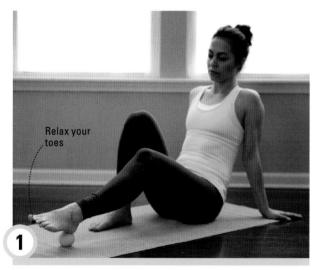

Relax your toes

1

Sit on the ground, place the ball beneath your left foot, and roll the area from the heel to the arch. If you find a painful point, massage it with circular movements for 20 to 30 seconds.

MODIFICATION

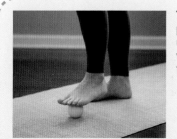

To increase pressure, stand upright and push your foot into the ball.

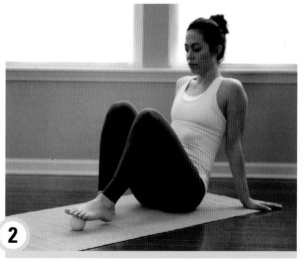

2

Refocus pressure and roll the area from the arch to the pads of the foot. Spend 20 to 30 seconds massaging any painful points. Then repeat for the right foot.

UPPER BODY
EXERCISES

SPINE RESTORATION

The thoracic spine runs from the neck to the lower back, and this release restores its length and flexibility. This part of the spine is crucial for movement of the head and shoulders, so doing this exercise regularly can alleviate neck and arm problems.

TARGETED MUSCLES

This exercise targets alignment of the thoracic spine vertebrae from the neck to the lower back. The torso bends and twists here.

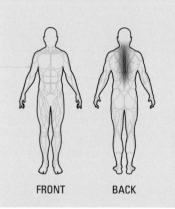

FRONT   BACK

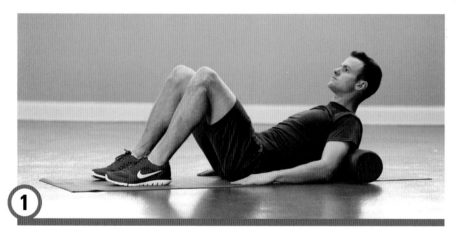

(1)

Lie with your back on the foam roller, and plant both feet on the ground for support.

CAUTION

To prevent spinal injury, stop immediately if you experience pain in your spine. Instead, attempt the modification for less pressure.

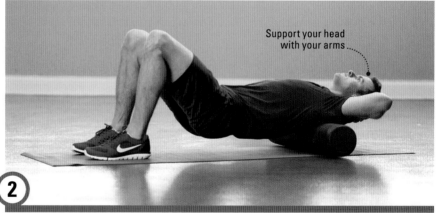

Support your head with your arms

(2)

Lift your hips off the ground by pushing through your feet, and inhale.

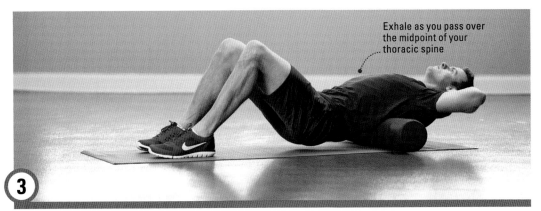

Exhale as you pass over the midpoint of your thoracic spine

3

Roll the length of your thoracic spine for 20 to 30 seconds, from the shoulder blades to the bottom of your ribcage, pushing and pulling with your legs.

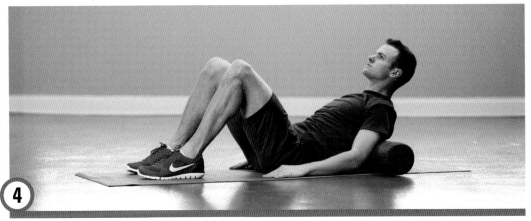

4

Pick three to four points during the movement to pause, drop your arms and hips to the ground, and exhale deeply while pushing into the roller.

MODIFICATIONS

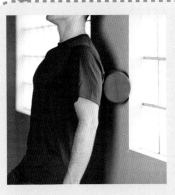

To decrease pressure, pin the roller against a wall and do slight squats to move it up and down.

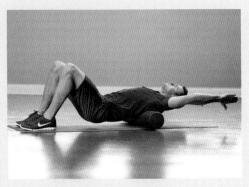

To make it harder, reach your arms straight above your head while rolling.

SPINE LENGTHENING

Lengthening your spine restores its natural curvature, from the base of the head to the hips. Your posture adapts to adverse lifestyle conditions, but this exercise can mitigate the discomfort. It's especially beneficial to perform before working out.

TARGETED MUSCLES

This exercise targets the core muscles in the back. These muscles align the spine to improve total body health.

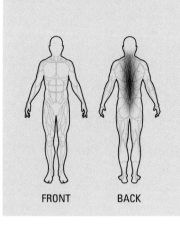

FRONT   BACK

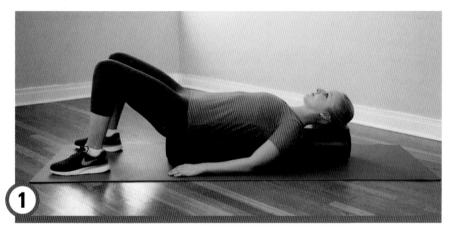

1

Lie with **your back** and head on the foam roller, and plant your feet on the ground for support. Rest your arms at your sides.

TIP

To achieve extra length in your spine, this exercise works well in combination with the Spine restoration and Hip flexor release exercises.

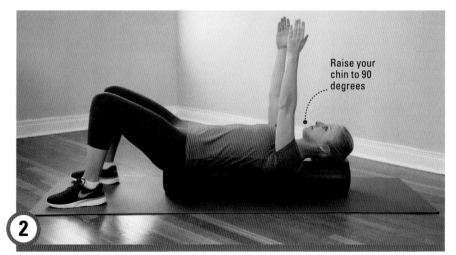

Raise your chin to 90 degrees

2

Inhale deeply through your nose and raise your arms straight up. Push your lower back into the roller.

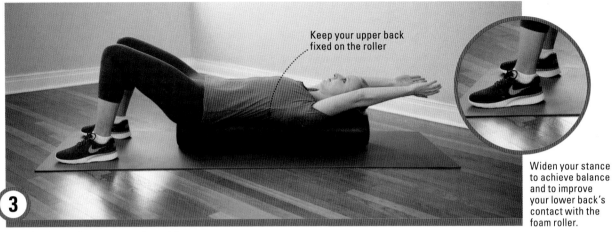

Keep your upper back
fixed on the roller

Widen your stance
to achieve balance
and to improve
your lower back's
contact with the
foam roller.

3

Exhale through your mouth and lower your
arms straight back to lengthen your spine.

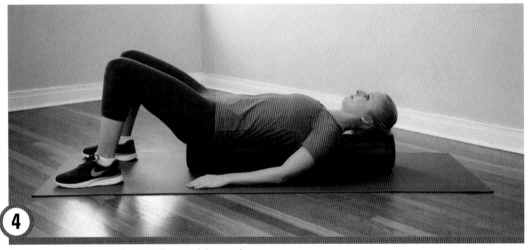

4

Return your arms to the starting position and
repeat the exercise 10 to 15 times.

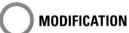

HOW IT HELPS

Pushing your lower
back into the roller
produces a contraction
in your abdominals,
making it a great
alternative way
to strengthen
the core.

MODIFICATION

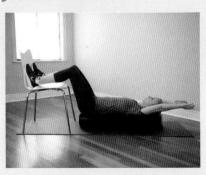

**To increase
pressure,** bend
your knees and
rest your feet on a
chair to maximize
contact with the
roller and to ease
hip tension.

LOWER BACK RELEASE

Foam rolling the lower back relieves the exhausted muscles that help stabilize the hips. These muscles straddle the lumbar spine and can become especially fatigued from poor posture or from running on uneven surfaces, slanted pavements, and trails.

TARGETED MUSCLES

This exercise targets the *quadratus lumborum*, a muscle that connects to the rib cage, pelvis, and spine as part of the body's core muscles. It helps support the spine and breathing.

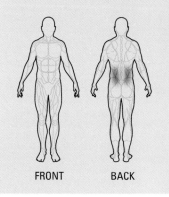

FRONT   BACK

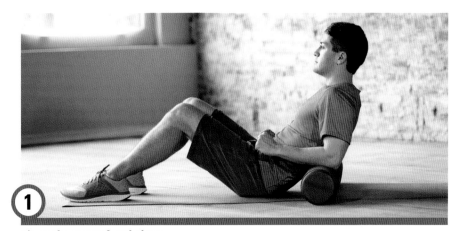

(1)

Sit on the ground and plant your feet in front of you. Position the foam roller behind your lower back.

CAUTION
To avoid damage and pain to your lumbar spine, you must only apply pressure to your muscles. Never foam-roll your bones.

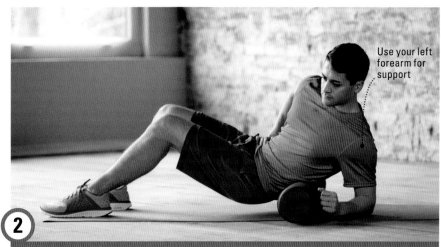

Use your left forearm for support

(2)

Turn your torso to the left, lift your hips, and apply pressure to the soft tissues on the left side of your spine, above the pelvis.

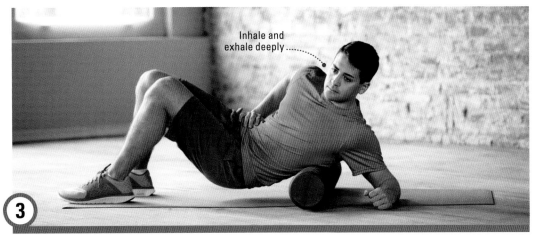

Inhale and
exhale deeply

3

Gently roll up and down over the length of your
lower back for 20 to 30 seconds.

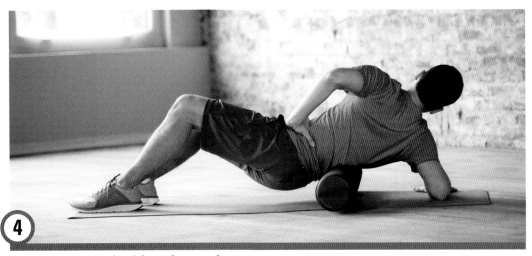

4

Turn your torso to the right and repeat the
exercise for your right lower back.

TIP
To diminish leg and hip
pain, do the exercise
often to strengthen
your legs and hips.
Weak legs require the
lower back to work
especially hard
during movement.

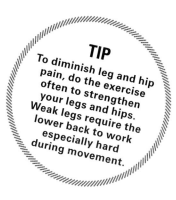

MODIFICATION

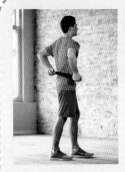

**To make it
easier,** use a
massage stick to
roll the soft tissue
next to your
lumbar spine.

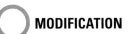

TARGETED LOWER BACK RELEASE

Foam rolling your lower back helps overall mobility, but targeting any knots best controls pain in the lumbar spine. These muscles strain easily due to inactive gluteals or during loaded twisting actions, such as turning and bending to pick up a child.

TARGETED MUSCLES

This exercise targets the *quadratus lumborum,* a muscle that connects to the rib cage, pelvis, and spine as part of the body's core musculature. It helps the body bend sideways.

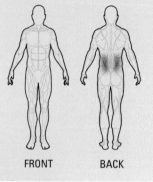

FRONT   BACK

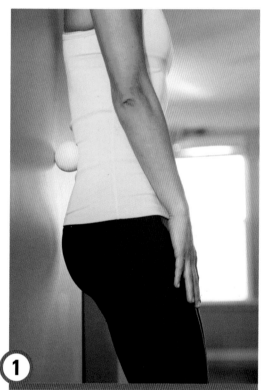

(1)

Stand upright and pin the ball between the wall and the area to the right of your spine, beneath the ribcage and above the pelvis.

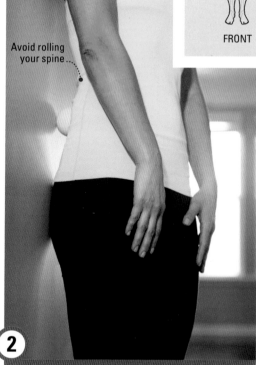

Avoid rolling your spine

(2)

Rotate to the right to roll the ball horizontally over the muscles from the spine to your side. If you find a painful point, massage it with circular movements for 20 to 30 seconds.

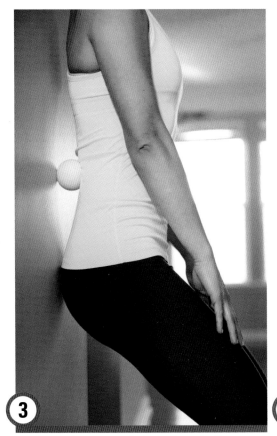

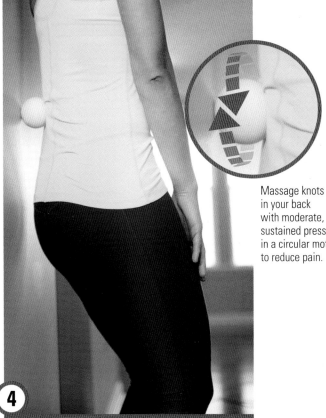

Massage knots in your back with moderate, sustained pressure in a circular motion to reduce pain.

3 **Bend your knees** to roll the ball vertically up your back, and spend 20 to 30 seconds massaging any particularly painful points.

4 **Rotate your body** to the left and repeat the exercise for the area to the left of your spine.

TIP
To permanently heal lower back pain, identify the cause. Releasing knots helps briefly, but weak muscles and bad habits chronically overwork the back.

MODIFICATION

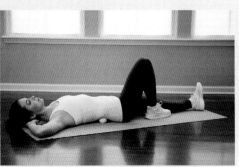

To increase pressure, lie on the ground and place the ball beneath your lower back.

MIDDLE BACK RELEASE

Massaging your middle back rebalances your head and shoulder area. If your head and arms are routinely pulled forwards during everyday activities, then your shoulders are likely to be overworked, and rolling the middle back reduces the tension and pain.

TARGETED MUSCLES

This exercise targets the *trapezius*, *rhomboids*, and *serratus posterior*, muscles that straddle the spine in the middle back. They support the head and shoulder blades.

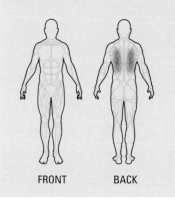

FRONT   BACK

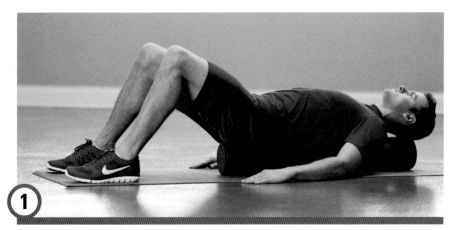

(1)

Lie with your back and head on the foam roller, and plant your feet on the ground for support.

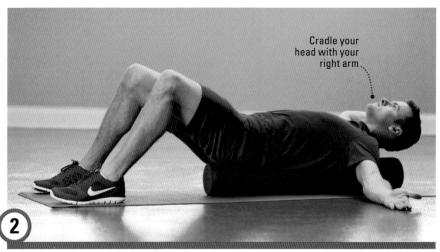

Cradle your head with your right arm

(2)

Rotate to the left to focus pressure on the muscles to the left of your spine, and extend your left arm along the ground.

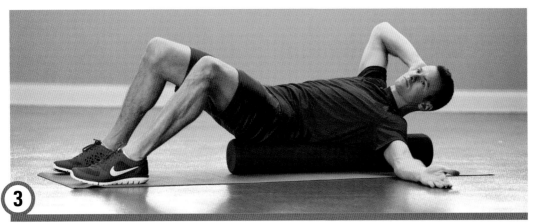

3 **Slowly roll from side to side,** from your shoulder blades to your spine, for 20 to 30 seconds. Use your legs and torso to propel your movement.

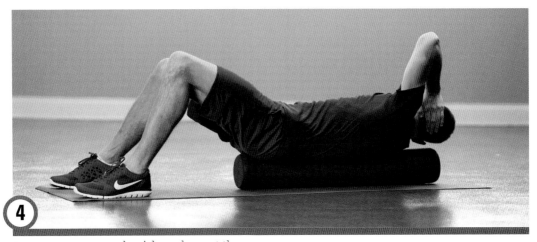

4 **Rotate your torso** to the right and repeat the exercise for your right middle back.

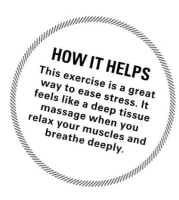

HOW IT HELPS

This exercise is a great way to ease stress. It feels like a deep tissue massage when you relax your muscles and breathe deeply.

MODIFICATION

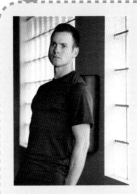

To make it easier, pin the roller against a wall with your back and lean into the roller.

TARGETED MIDDLE BACK RELEASE

Painful knots often afflict the middle back. Lifting heavy objects, over-exercising, and poor posture cause deviations from your neutral spinal alignment, causing the painful points. Do this easy exercise frequently to alleviate your discomfort.

TARGETED MUSCLES

This exercise targets the superficial muscles of the middle back (those closest to the surface). They straddle the vertebrae to protect and align the spine.

FRONT   BACK

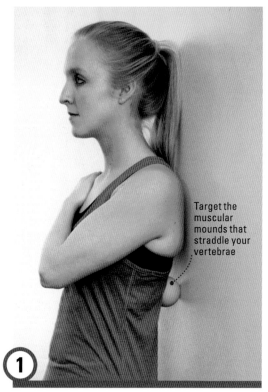

Target the muscular mounds that straddle your vertebrae

1

Stand upright and pin the ball between the wall and the area to the left of your spine below the shoulder blade. Cross your left arm over your chest and lean into the ball.

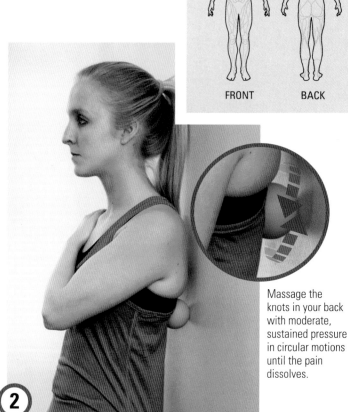

Massage the knots in your back with moderate, sustained pressure in circular motions until the pain dissolves.

2

Bend your knees to roll the ball up your middle back. If you find a painful point, massage it with circular movements for 20 to 30 seconds.

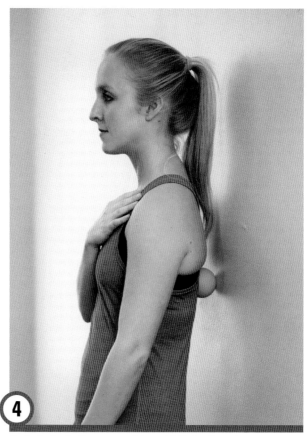

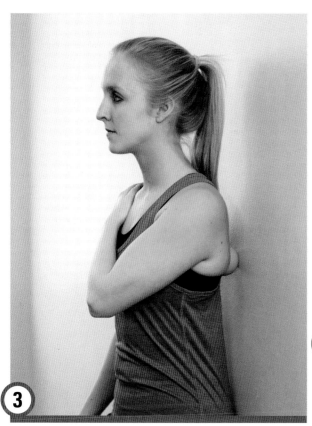

4

Switch the ball to your right middle back and repeat the exercise.

3

Rotate your torso to the right and refocus pressure closer to your spine. Spend 20 to 30 seconds massaging any particularly painful points.

HOW IT HELPS
This release alleviates referred pain in the back and lower body. Target these knots when you have lower back, gluteal, and leg pain.

○ **MODIFICATION**

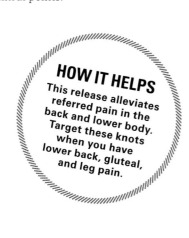

To make it easier, place the ball in a long sock and hold it over the top of your shoulder.

MIDDLE BACK ACTIVATION

This simple exercise restores balance to taut back muscles, which impact the shoulder area. Inactivity in your middle back leads to an overactive upper back, causing soreness in the neck, shoulders, and arms. This is common in people who reach forwards often.

TARGETED MUSCLES

This exercise targets the *trapezius*, the diamond-shaped muscle travelling from the base of the neck out to the shoulders and in towards the lower back. It supports the shoulder blades and arms.

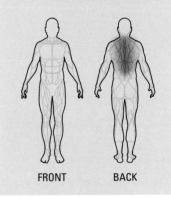

FRONT   BACK

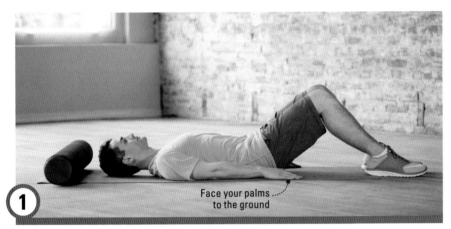

Face your palms to the ground

①

Lie on your back and plant your feet on the ground. Place the foam roller above your head.

TIP

To depress (move down) the shoulder blades for an effective starting position, stretch your hands down to your feet before you begin each repetition.

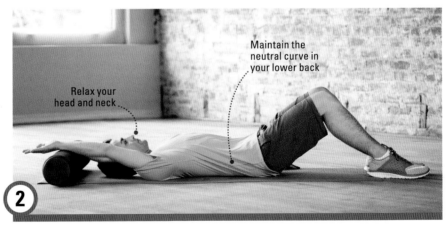

Relax your head and neck

Maintain the neutral curve in your lower back

②

Lift your right arm straight up and back in an arc. When your arm makes contact with the roller, press it further into the roller until your middle back contracts, and hold for 3 seconds.

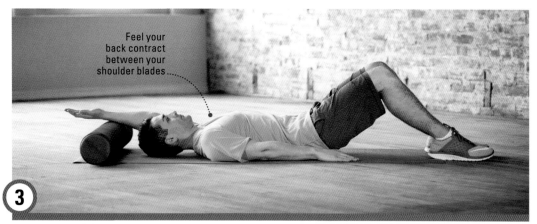

Feel your back contract between your shoulder blades...

3

Return your right arm to the starting position, and repeat the arcing motion with your left arm.

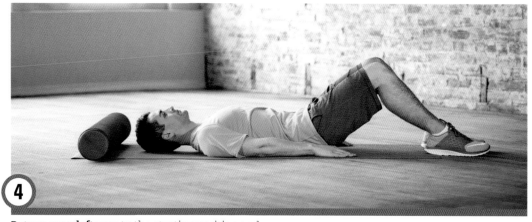

4

Return your left arm to the starting position and repeat the exercise 10 times.

⭕ MODIFICATIONS

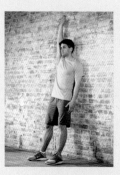

To make it easier, lean back against a wall and raise your arms up to the wall above your head.

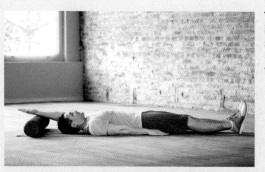

To make it harder, straighten your legs to challenge your lower back.

TARGETED SHOULDER RELEASE

Different jobs or activities that require you to repeatedly reach back, up, or out can overwork your shoulders. These actions cause knots and referred pain throughout the upper body, but doing this exercise relieves tension and improves flexibility.

TARGETED MUSCLES

This release targets the three distinct regions of the deltoid: anterior deltoid, lateral deltoid, and posterior deltoid. They control reaching movements.

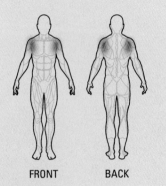

FRONT   BACK

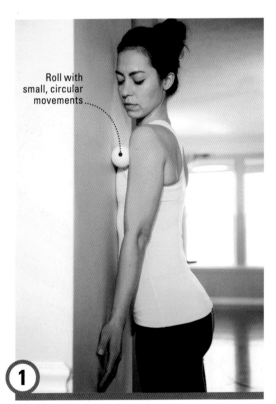

Roll with small, circular movements

①

Stand upright and pin the ball between the wall and the front of your left shoulder. Roll the front of your shoulder for about 25 seconds.

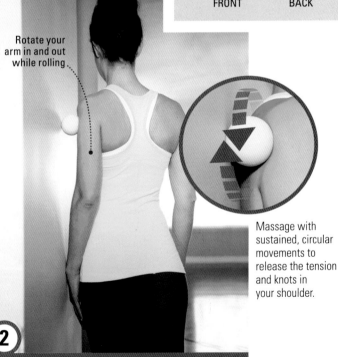

Rotate your arm in and out while rolling

Massage with sustained, circular movements to release the tension and knots in your shoulder.

②

Turn your body to roll the side of your left shoulder for 20 to 30 seconds.

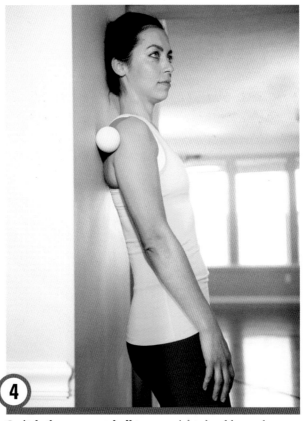

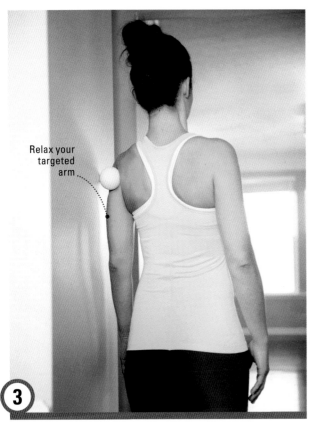

Relax your
targeted
arm

3

Turn your body again to roll the back of your left
shoulder for 20 to 30 seconds.

4

Switch the massage ball to your right shoulder and
repeat the exercise.

TIP
To treat incessant
pain, even while at
rest, look for any
knots in surrounding
muscles; knots in the
pectorals or underarms
can refer pain to
the shoulders.

MODIFICATION

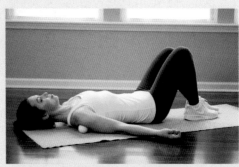

To increase pressure, lie on the ground and
place the ball beneath your shoulder.

SHOULDER BLADE RELEASE

The shoulder blades mobilize several movements, so the many attached muscles can become temperamental and overworked. If you always hold your arms in front of you – typing or on your phone – you can benefit from this lengthening exercise.

TARGETED MUSCLES

This exercise targets the rotator cuff muscles: the *infraspinatus*, *supraspinatus*, and *teres minor*. They stabilize the shoulders.

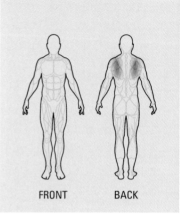

FRONT   BACK

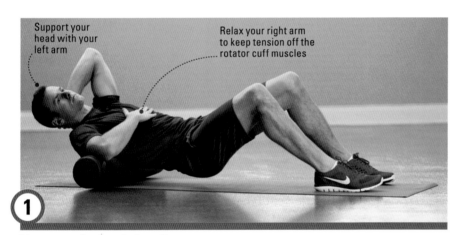

Support your head with your left arm

Relax your right arm to keep tension off the rotator cuff muscles

1

Lie on your back and place the foam roller beneath your right shoulder. Plant both feet on the ground, raise your hips, and rotate your torso to the right.

TIP

For permanently pain-free shoulders, determine the cause and adjust bad habits. For example, pull the keyboard closer to you when typing.

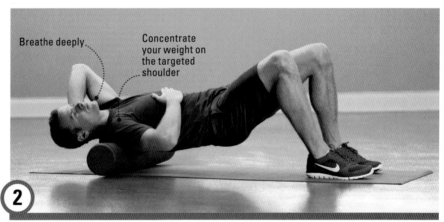

Breathe deeply

Concentrate your weight on the targeted shoulder

2

Roll back and forth over your right shoulder blade for 20 to 30 seconds, pushing and pulling with your legs. Then rotate your torso to the left and repeat the exercise for your left shoulder.

FRONT SHOULDER RELEASE

Releasing the front of your shoulder restores healthy movement in your arm and alleviates any pain in surrounding areas. Players of overhead sports such as basketball, netball, and volleyball especially benefit from improved flexibility by doing this exercise.

TARGETED MUSCLES

This exercise targets the anterior deltoid in the front of the shoulders. This part of the deltoid lifts the arm away from the body.

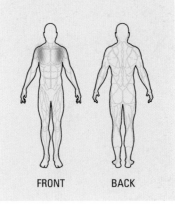

FRONT   BACK

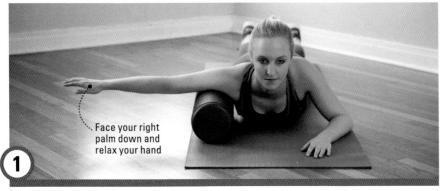

Face your right palm down and relax your hand

1

Lie on your stomach and extend your right arm 90 degrees. Place the foam roller beneath the front of your right shoulder.

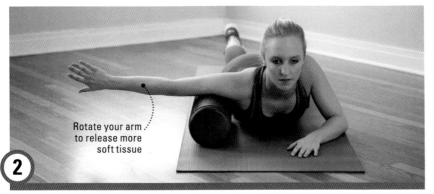

Rotate your arm to release more soft tissue

2

Roll your upper body from side to side to roll the width of your right shoulder for 20 to 30 seconds. Then switch the foam roller to your left shoulder and repeat the exercise.

MODIFICATION

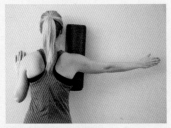

To decrease pressure, extend your arm and pin the foam roller between the wall and your front shoulder.

SHOULDER BLADE MOBILIZATION

For more effective pushing and pulling and a healthier rotator cuff, use this exercise to develop shoulder blade stability and mobility. A stable shoulder blade produces efficient protraction and retraction and helps alleviate shoulder, back, and neck pain.

TARGETED MUSCLES

This exercise targets the *serratus anterior* (beneath the shoulder blade) and the rhomboid (between the shoulder blade and spine). They stabilize the shoulder blades.

FRONT   BACK

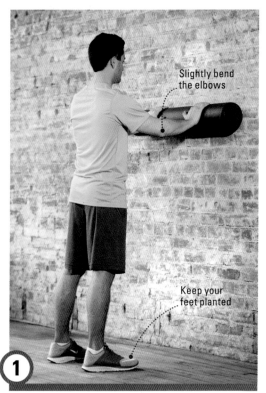

Slightly bend the elbows

Keep your feet planted

1 **Pin the foam roller to the wall** with your hands at shoulder height. Extend your arms. Lean forwards.

Keep your head raised

2 **Retract, or draw, your shoulder blades together,** so that you move slightly towards the wall.

To improve the stability of your shoulder joints, keep your hands fixed and upright on the roller.

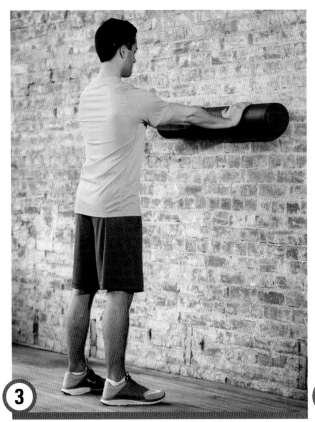

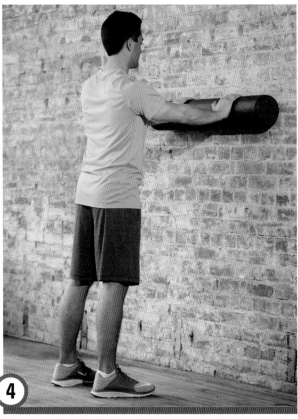

3 **Protract, or pull your shoulder blades apart,** so that you move away from the wall. At the same time, rotate your elbows in and hold for 2 seconds.

4 **Return to the starting position** and repeat the same exercise 10 times.

MODIFICATIONS

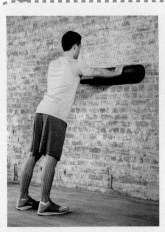

To increase pressure, plant your feet farther from the wall.

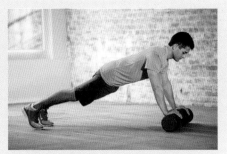

To make it harder, do the exercise from a push-up position on the ground.

CHEST RELEASE

Tension in one muscle group can refer pain to the opposing muscle group, so a tight chest can cause knots to form in the upper back and shoulders, for example. Use this exercise to restore circulation and reduce referred pain in your upper body.

TARGETED MUSCLES

This exercise targets the *pectoralis major* and *pectoralis minor* of the chest. These muscles pull the arms forwards.

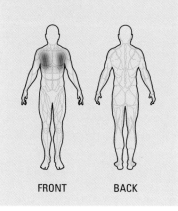

FRONT   BACK

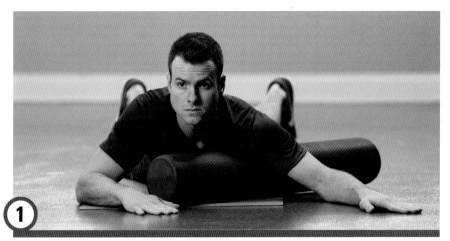

1

Lie on your stomach and extend your left arm along the ground. Place the foam roller beneath your left underarm.

TIP
To make the exercise easier, you can use your opposite hand to turn the roller and facilitate the movement.

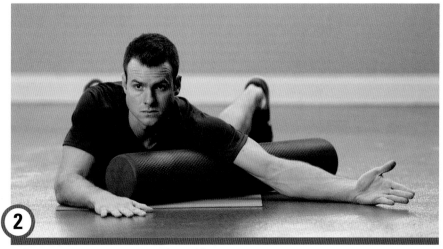

2

Roll up to your upper arm, pulling with your feet, and rotate your palm up.

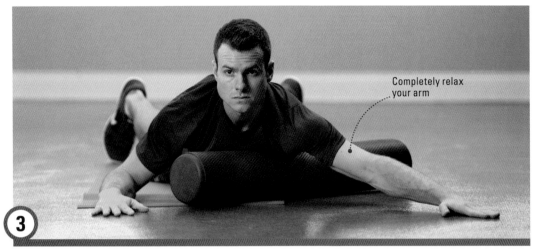

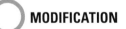
Completely relax your arm

3

Roll down to your sternum and rotate your palm down. Continue to roll the shoulder and chest area for 20 to 30 seconds.

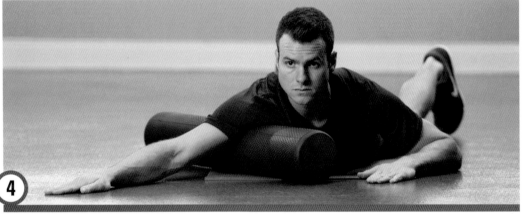

4

Switch the foam roller to your right underarm and repeat the exercise.

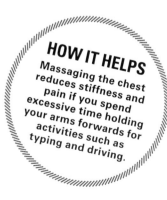
HOW IT HELPS
Massaging the chest reduces stiffness and pain if you spend excessive time holding your arms forwards for activities such as typing and driving.

MODIFICATION

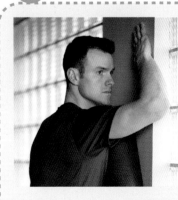

To make it easier, pin the roller to a wall with your chest.

TARGETED CHEST RELEASE

If you have a desk job, your chest may have quite a few knots. Prolonged sitting pulls your shoulders forwards, which shortens your chest muscles and causes pain. Using a ball to release the muscles will alleviate soreness and improve flexibility.

TARGETED MUSCLES

This release targets the *pectoralis major* and *pectoralis minor* in the chest. These pull and rotate the arms toward the body's centre.

FRONT   BACK

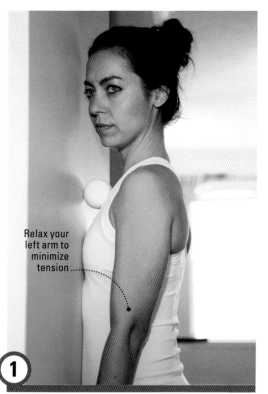

Relax your left arm to minimize tension

①

Stand upright and pin the ball between the wall and your left pectoral region beneath the collarbone. Lean into the ball.

The ball will move only slightly with this shift

Sustained massage and moderate pressure to this area make the chest feel looser and breathing easier.

②

Shift from side to side to roll the ball across your upper chest. If you find a painful point, massage it with circular movements for 20 to 30 seconds.

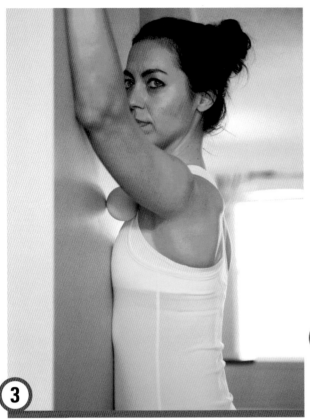

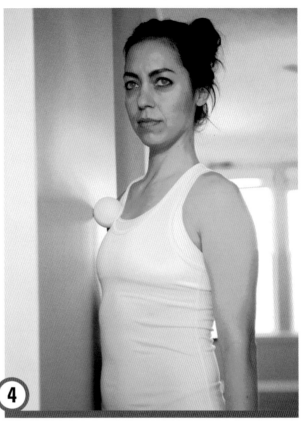

④ Switch the ball across to your right side and repeat the exercise.

③ Move the ball to your lower chest and raise your left arm. Shift from side to side to roll the ball across your lower chest, and spend 20 to 30 seconds massaging particularly painful points.

HOW IT HELPS
This release soothes upper body pain if you carry a large bag or backpack. But for a permanent solution, you must actively change your habits.

MODIFICATION

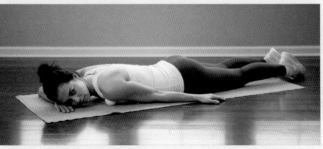

To access other trigger points, lie on the ground, place the ball beneath your chest, and slowly arc your arm.

LATS RELEASE

To alleviate tension in and around your shoulders, the Lats release elongates the muscles and restores overhead function. If you lift overhead or hold your arms at your side for extended periods, you'll benefit from massaging this area of your back.

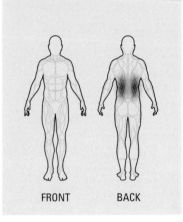
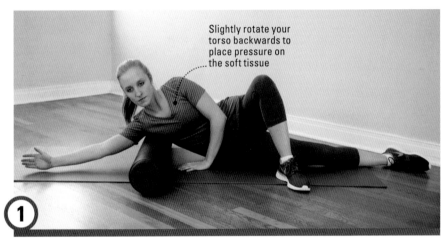

Slightly rotate your torso backwards to place pressure on the soft tissue

1

Lie on your right side, place the foam roller beneath your right underarm, and plant your left foot on the ground for support.

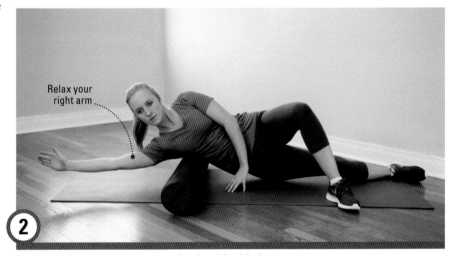

Relax your right arm

2

Lift your hips and roll down to the shoulder blade, pushing with your left arm and leg.

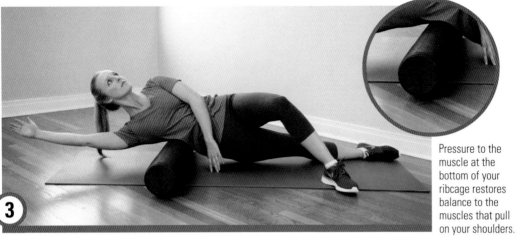

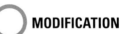

Pressure to the muscle at the bottom of your ribcage restores balance to the muscles that pull on your shoulders.

3

Rotate your torso back and roll to the bottom of your ribcage. Continue to roll the length of your right lat for 20 to 30 seconds.

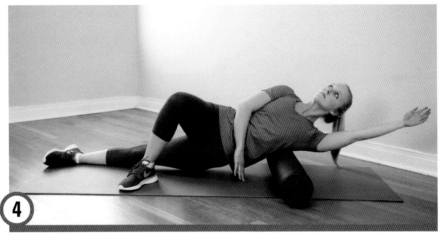

4

Switch the foam roller to your left side and repeat the exercise.

TIP

To follow the lat muscle, which wraps around your back and side, rotate your ribcage forwards and backwards as you roll.

MODIFICATION

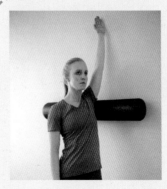

To make it easier, extend your arm along a wall, pin the roller to the wall with your side, and bend your knees to move the roller.

UNDERARM RELEASE

The small movement of this exercise targets the area where the arms join the ribcage. If you keep your arms close to your sides a lot, these muscles can become taut and painful, but foam rolling the underarm can restore length and circulation.

TARGETED MUSCLES

This exercise targets the *infraspinatus*, *teres major,* and *teres minor,* the muscles in the underarms. They help stabilize the humerus (upper-arm bone).

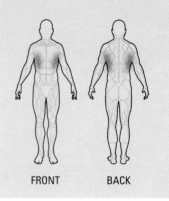

FRONT   BACK

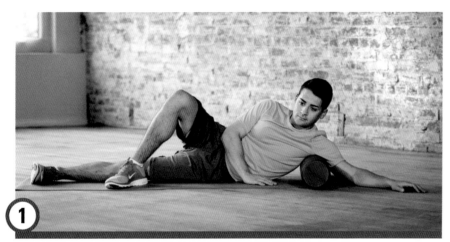

①

Lie on your left side, place the foam roller beneath your left underarm, and plant your right foot on the ground for support.

Use your right arm to facilitate the rotation of your torso or the movement of the foam roller.

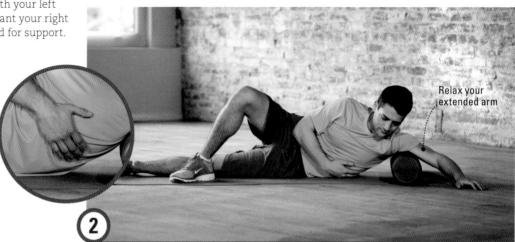

Relax your extended arm

②

Rotate your torso forwards and roll up to your upper arm, pulling with your right foot.

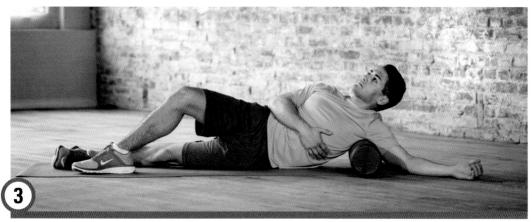

3

Rotate your torso and left arm back and roll to the bottom of your underarm. Continue to roll the length of your underarm for 20 to 30 seconds.

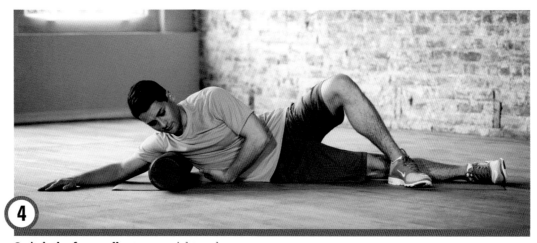

4

Switch the foam roller to your right underarm and repeat the exercise.

HOW IT HELPS

This release restores balance in the shoulder complex by increasing flexibility in certain muscles and decreasing tension in opposing muscles.

MODIFICATION

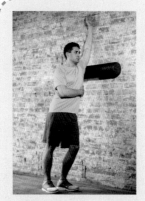

To make it easier, extend your arm along a wall and pin the roller to the wall with your underarm.

BICEPS RELEASE

If you hold heavy objects with a flexed elbow, you may develop pain in your biceps. Massage this muscle group to improve circulation and alleviate tension. You can trace many disorders of the hand, wrist, elbow, and shoulder to chronically tight biceps.

TARGETED MUSCLES

This exercise targets the biceps muscle group, located in the inner upper arm. These muscles help flex the elbows, rotate the forearms, and stabilize the shoulder blades.

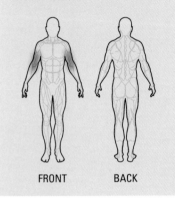

FRONT   BACK

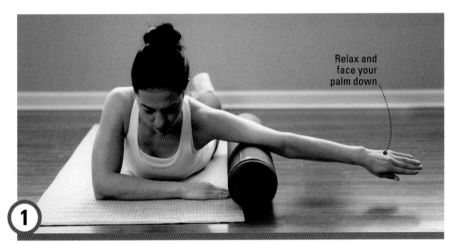

Relax and face your palm down

(1)

Lie on your stomach and extend your left arm to 90 degrees. Place the foam roller beneath your left biceps.

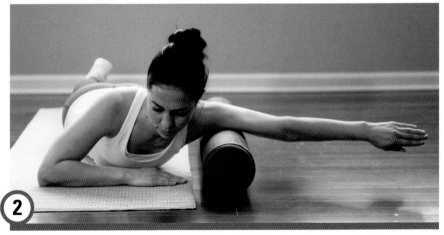

(2)

Shift your upper body from side to side to roll the length of your left biceps for 20 to 30 seconds, from your shoulder to your elbow.

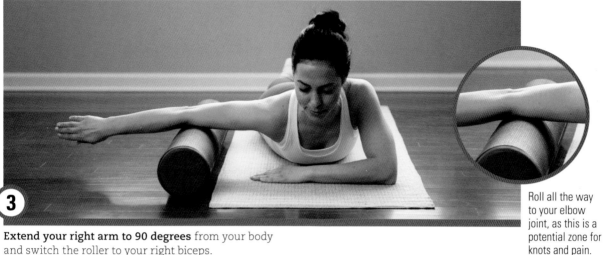

3

Extend your right arm to 90 degrees from your body
and switch the roller to your right biceps.

Roll all the way
to your elbow
joint, as this is a
potential zone for
knots and pain.

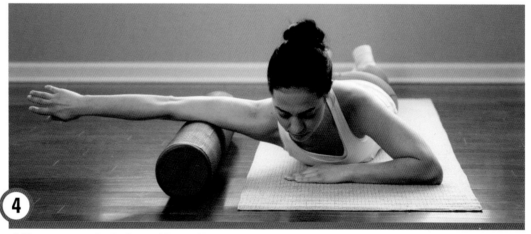
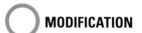

4

Shift your upper body from side to side to roll
the length of your right biceps for 20 to 30
seconds, from your shoulder to your elbow.

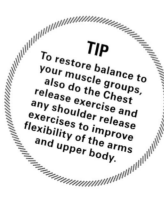

TIP
To restore balance to
your muscle groups,
also do the Chest
release exercise and
any shoulder release
exercises to improve
flexibility of the arms
and upper body.

MODIFICATION

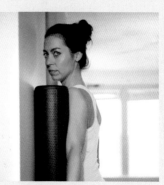

**To make it
easier,** pin the
foam roller to
the wall with
your biceps.

TRICEPS RELEASE

For elbow and shoulder pain, the Triceps release can relieve referred pain. Repetitively extending the elbow joint, whether at your job or while playing a sport, can burden your triceps with sensitive and painful knots that the foam roller can release.

TARGETED MUSCLES

This exercise targets the triceps muscles, located in the back of the upper arms. They extend the elbows and stabilize the shoulders.

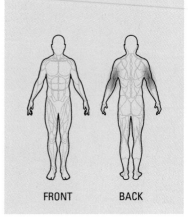

FRONT   BACK

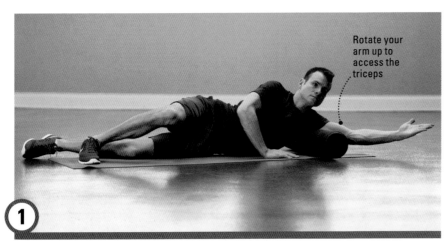

Rotate your arm up to access the triceps

1

Lie on your left side, place the foam roller beneath your left arm, and plant your right foot on the ground for support.

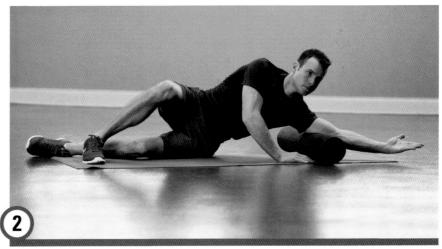

2

Roll down to your elbow joint, pushing with your right arm and right leg.

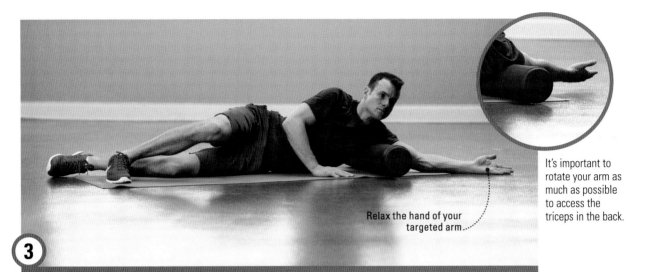

It's important to rotate your arm as much as possible to access the triceps in the back.

Relax the hand of your targeted arm...

3

Roll up to your underarm. Continue to roll the length of the triceps for 20 to 30 seconds.

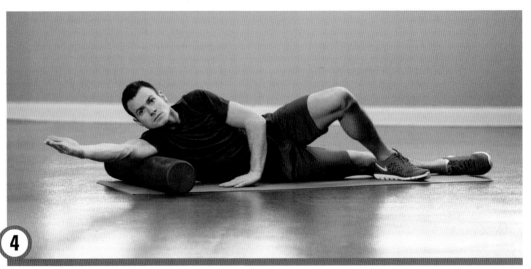

4

Switch the foam roller to your right triceps and repeat the exercise.

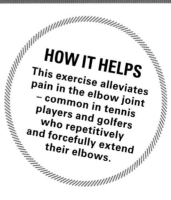

HOW IT HELPS
This exercise alleviates pain in the elbow joint – common in tennis players and golfers who repetitively and forcefully extend their elbows.

FOREARM WALL SLIDE

This wall slide establishes shoulder mobility in an overhead position. If you load your shoulder joint for activities such as painting a wall or putting luggage in an overhead compartment, then mobilize your shoulders so you're not vulnerable to injury.

TARGETED MUSCLES

This exercise targets the *serratus anterior* (located along the sides of the ribcage). This muscle rotates the shoulder blades upwards.

FRONT   BACK

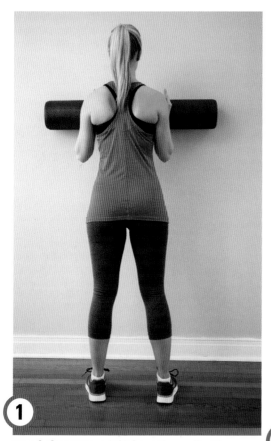

1 **Stand about 31cm (1ft) from the wall** with your feet shoulder-width apart. Pin the foam roller to the wall with the sides of your hands.

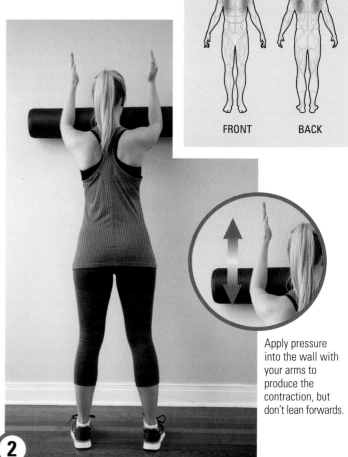

Apply pressure into the wall with your arms to produce the contraction, but don't lean forwards.

2 **Apply pressure into the roller** through your hands. Slowly glide your forearms up over the roller without raising your shoulders.

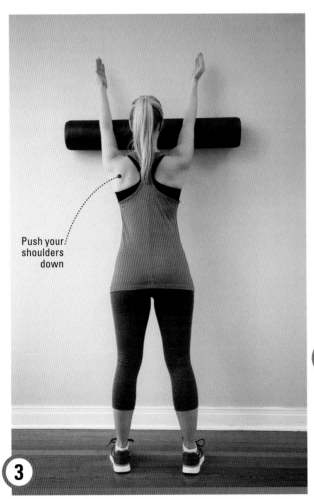

Push your
shoulders
down

3

Rotate your palms in as you move up. Continue to glide
up until you fully extend your arms.

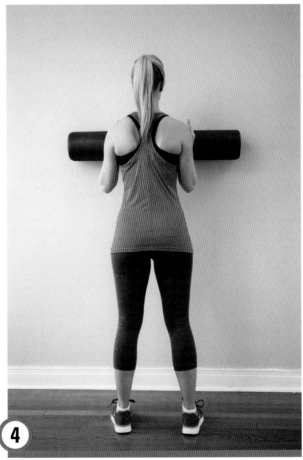

4

Return your arms to the starting position and repeat
the exercise 10 times.

TIP
To target the correct
muscle, begin by
drawing your shoulder
blades together. The
key is to slide as high
as you can without
lifting your shoulders.

NECK RELEASE

Rolling the back of the neck helps if you habitually look down. A chronic forward head position overworks the muscles in the base of the skull, but rolling the back of the neck helps to alleviate the tension and even reduce the occurrence of headaches.

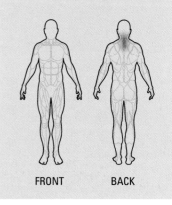
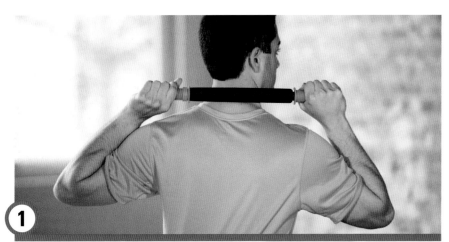

1

Stand comfortably and hold the massage stick against the right side of your neck.

Firmly hold the stick and push forwards to produce a moderate amount of pressure.

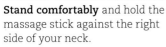

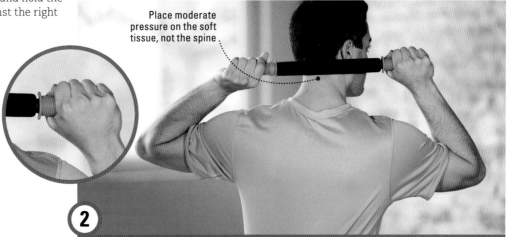

Place moderate pressure on the soft tissue, not the spine

2

Turn your head to the right and roll up the right side of your neck to your ear.

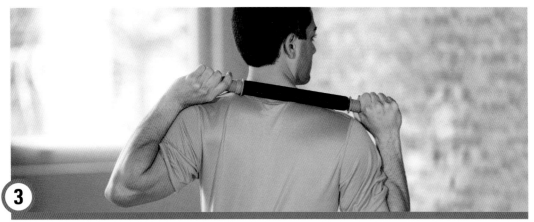

3

Roll down the right side of your neck to your shoulders. Continue to roll the length of the right side of your neck for 20 to 30 seconds.

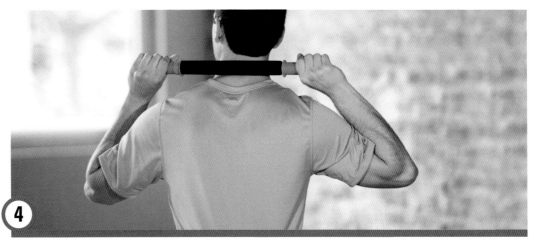

4

Turn your head to the left and repeat the exercise for the left side of your neck.

HOW IT HELPS
This exercise reduces tension from "text neck" if you habitually look down at a phone. Try using your eye muscles instead of the neck to look down.

MODIFICATION

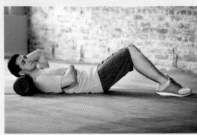

To make it easier, place a foam roller beneath your neck and slowly turn your head from side to side.

FINGER FLEXOR RELEASE

You use your network of hand and finger flexors whenever you carry a bag, type, or shake hands. They pull your hand and fingers inwards, but over- and underuse can cause tightness. Use this exercise to reduce the pain and tension.

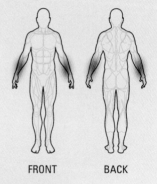

TARGETED MUSCLES

This exercise targets the hand and finger flexors, which originate near the inside of the elbow. They bend the hand inwards and clench the fingers and thumb.

FRONT   BACK

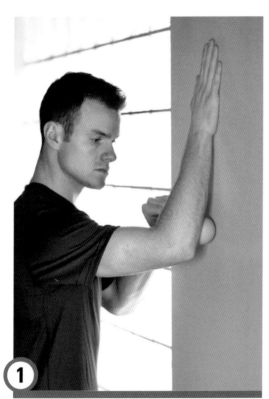

1

Pin the ball between the wall and the inside of your right forearm, flatten your palm against the wall, and lean into the ball.

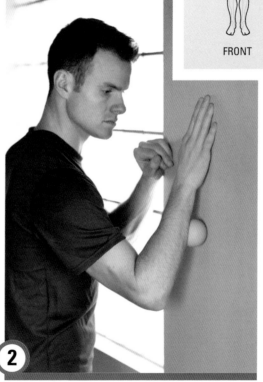

2

Move the right forearm up to roll the ball over the flexors. If you find a painful point, massage it with circular movements for 20 to 30 seconds. Then repeat the exercise for your left arm.

FINGER EXTENSOR RELEASE

When you straighten, lift, stretch, or point your fingers, you use your hand and finger extensors. These are prone to overuse and injury, especially if you type on a misplaced keyboard with your wrists lower than the keys. Perform this exercise to relieve pain.

TARGETED MUSCLES

This exercise targets the hand and finger extensors, which originate near the outside of the elbows. They bend the hands backwards and lift the fingers and thumbs.

FRONT   BACK

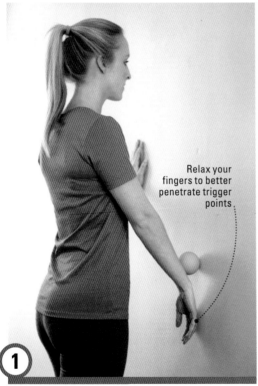

Relax your fingers to better penetrate trigger points

1 **Pin the ball** between the wall and the outside of your right forearm. Lean into the ball.

2 **Bend your knees** to roll the ball over the extensors. If you find a painful point, massage it with circular movements for 20 to 30 seconds. Then repeat the exercise for your left arm.

TARGETED PALM RELEASE

You use your hands for almost every activity during the day, from writing to grasping a bag. You can easily overwork the muscles in your palm, so do this exercise frequently as a simple cure for any knots and tension in your hands.

TARGETED MUSCLES

This release targets the four largest muscles in the hand. They control movements of the thumb.

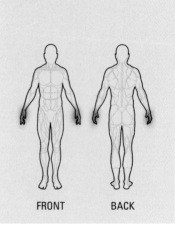

FRONT   BACK

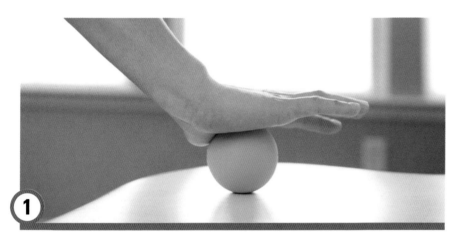

1

Place the ball on an elevated surface and rest your right palm on the ball.

HOW IT HELPS
Rolling the hands stimulates the nerves in your skin to send information to your body to improve your coordination.

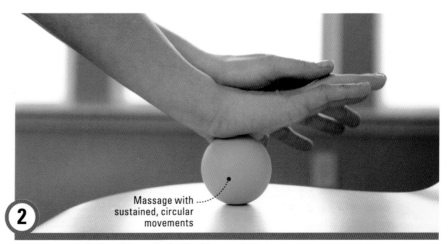

Massage with sustained, circular movements

2

Press your right hand into the ball with your left hand and massage the area between your palm and thumb for 20 to 30 seconds.

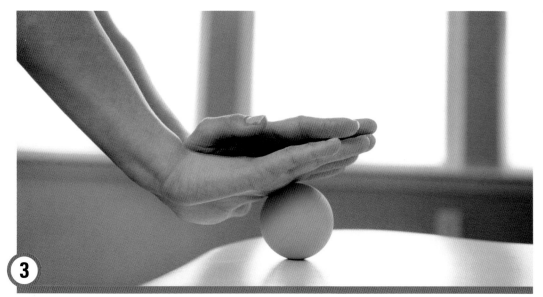

3

Glide the rest of your palm over the ball. If you find
a particularly painful point, massage it with circular
movements for 20 to 30 seconds.

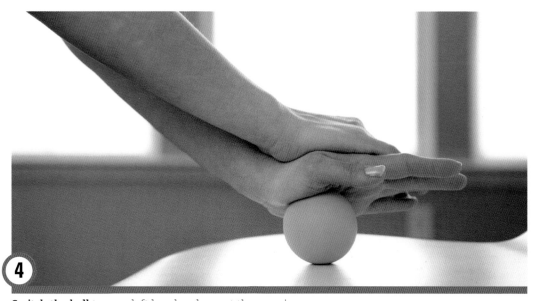

4

Switch the ball to your left hand and repeat the exercise.

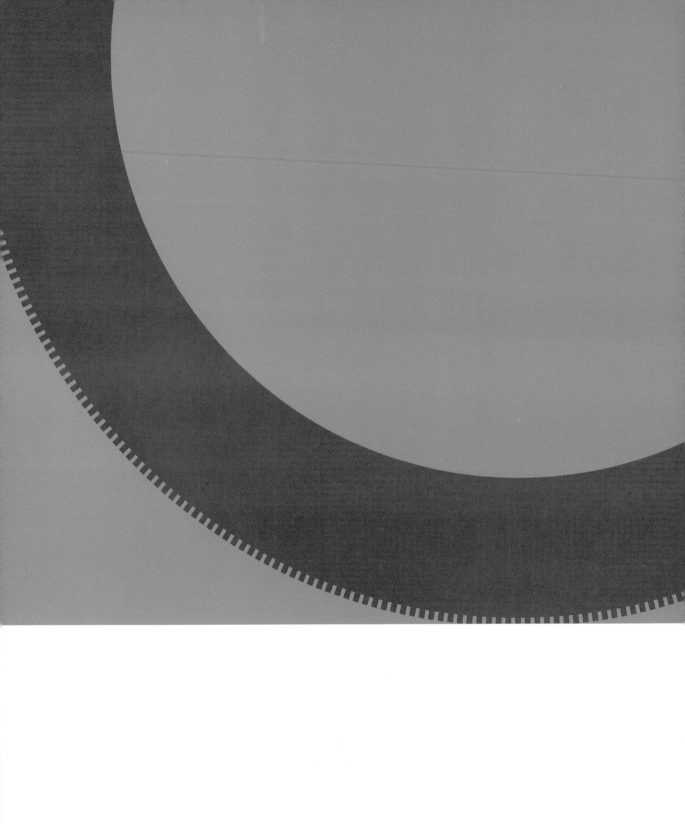

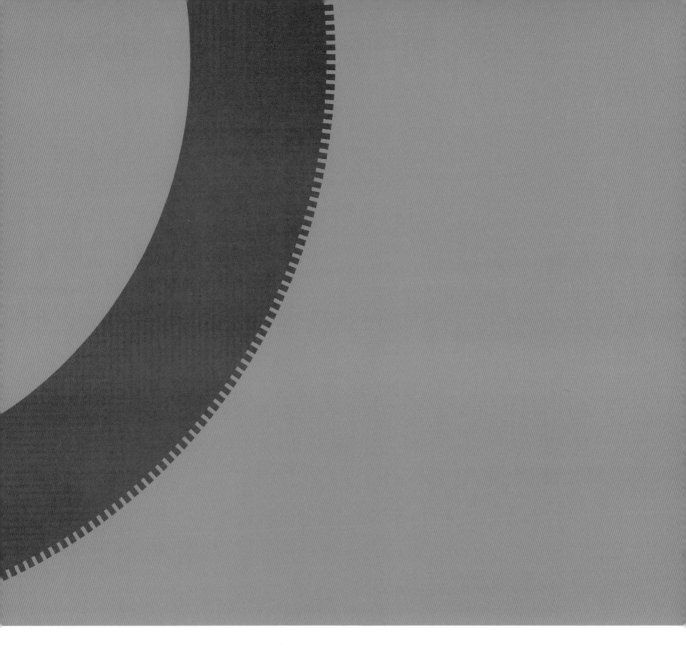

PAIN RELIEF PROGRAMMES

UPPER BACK

Reaching to a keyboard or looking down at a mobile phone strains the upper back, as certain muscles become overworked and others underworked. To reduce pain, do these exercises to improve your back's strength and flexibility.

WHAT YOU NEED

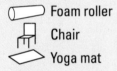

Foam roller

Chair

Yoga mat

WHAT TO DO

- Do the exercises in order.
- Spend 30 to 45 seconds on each exercise.
- Breathe deeply and relax your muscles.
- Devote extra time to releasing more painful upper body muscles.

	EXERCISE	TOOL	PAGE
1	CHEST RELEASE		P118
2	FRONT SHOULDER RELEASE		P115
3	SPINE RESTORATION		P98
4	SPINE LENGTHENING		P100
5	SITTING RIBCAGE ROTATION		P34
6	MIDDLE BACK ACTIVATION		P110
7	PLANK PROGRESSIONS		P24

SPINE LENGTHENING

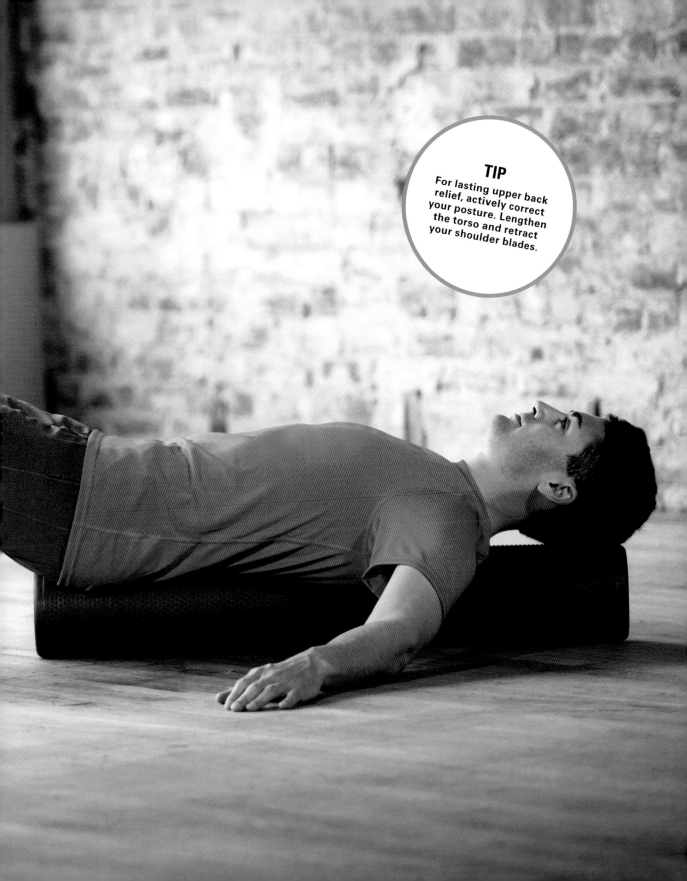

TIP
For lasting upper back relief, actively correct your posture. Lengthen the torso and retract your shoulder blades.

LOWER BACK

When your hips are immobile or tight, the lower back compensates, causing knots and poor alignment. Perform this programme to activate your hip muscles, massage the related muscles, and relieve lower back discomfort.

WHAT YOU NEED

Foam roller

Massage ball

Yoga mat

WHAT TO DO

- Do the exercises in order.
- Spend 30 to 45 seconds on each exercise.
- Monitor your pain level and adjust the pressure accordingly.
- Focus pressure on your soft tissue and avoid rolling bones.

	EXERCISE	TOOL	PAGE
1	HIP FLEXOR RELEASE		P50
2	HAMSTRINGS RELEASE		P72
3	SPINE RESTORATION		P98
4	LOWER BACK RELEASE		P102
5	TARGETED LOWER BACK RELEASE		P104
6	SPINE LENGTHENING		P100
7	BIRD DOG REACH		P30

LOWER BACK RELEASE ▶

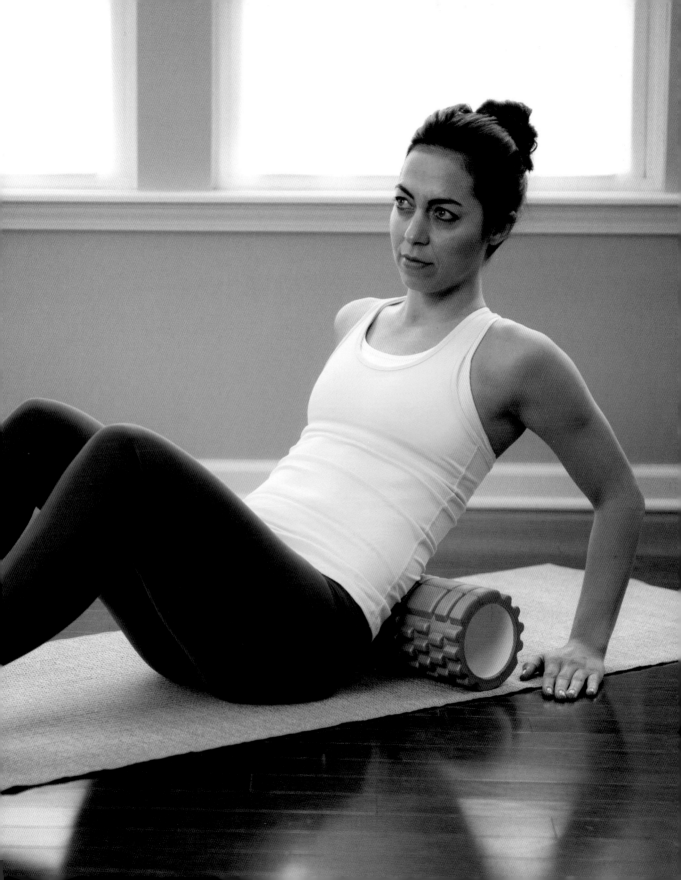

SHOULDER AND NECK

Joints and soft tissues in your neck and shoulders strain easily if you frequently use your arms to reach overheads and forwards, you have poor posture, or you rarely use your upper body during the day. Do these exercises to subdue the pain.

EXERCISE		TOOL	PAGE
1	**NECK RELEASE**		**P132**
2	**SHOULDER BLADE RELEASE**		**P114**
3	**SPINE LENGTHENING**		**P100**
4	**CHEST RELEASE**		**P118**
5	**MIDDLE BACK RELEASE**		**P106**

WHAT YOU NEED

Massage stick
Foam roller
Yoga mat

WHAT TO DO

- Do the exercises in order.
- Spend 30 to 45 seconds on each exercise.
- Monitor your pain level and adjust the pressure accordingly.
- Relax your neck and arm muscles so you're more receptive to release.

SHOULDER BLADE RELEASE ▶

TARGETED SHOULDER AND NECK

If you have sharp pain or tightness in the shoulders or neck, you tend to have many over- and underused muscles that refer pain through the area. Perform this programme to relieve the knots and ensure pain-free posture.

WHAT YOU NEED

- ○ Massage ball
- ⬭ Foam roller
- ▱ Yoga mat

WHAT TO DO

- o Do the exercises in order.
- o Spend 30 to 45 seconds on each exercise.
- o Breathe deeply and relax your muscles.
- o Find the knots that refer pain through your shoulders and neck.

	EXERCISE	TOOL	PAGE
1	**TARGETED MIDDLE BACK RELEASE**	○	P**108**
2	**TARGETED SHOULDER RELEASE**	○	P**112**
3	**SHOULDER BLADE RELEASE**	⬭	P**114**
4	**TARGETED CHEST RELEASE**	○	P**120**
5	**UNDERARM RELEASE**	⬭	P**124**

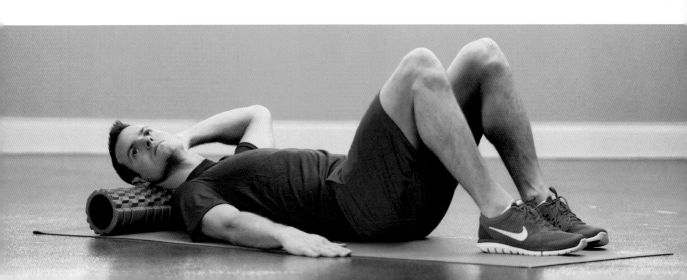

HIPS

Several muscles originate and end around the pelvis, making your hips prone to tightness and pain. Use this programme to improve flexibility and muscle health if your hips and related muscles are overworked or underused.

WHAT YOU NEED

- Foam roller
- Massage ball
- Yoga mat

WHAT TO DO

- Do the exercises in order.
- Spend 30 to 45 seconds on each exercise.
- Breathe deeply and relax your muscles.
- Repeat the exercises that target your most tense muscles.

	EXERCISE	TOOL	PAGE
1	HIP FLEXOR RELEASE		P50
2	GLUTEAL GROUP RELEASE		P58
3	QUADRICEPS RELEASE		P66
4	OUTER THIGH AND HIP RELEASE		P70
5	INNER THIGH RELEASE		P76
6	HAMSTRINGS RELEASE		P72
7	TARGETED HIP ROTATOR RELEASE		P52

OUTER THIGH AND HIP RELEASE ▶

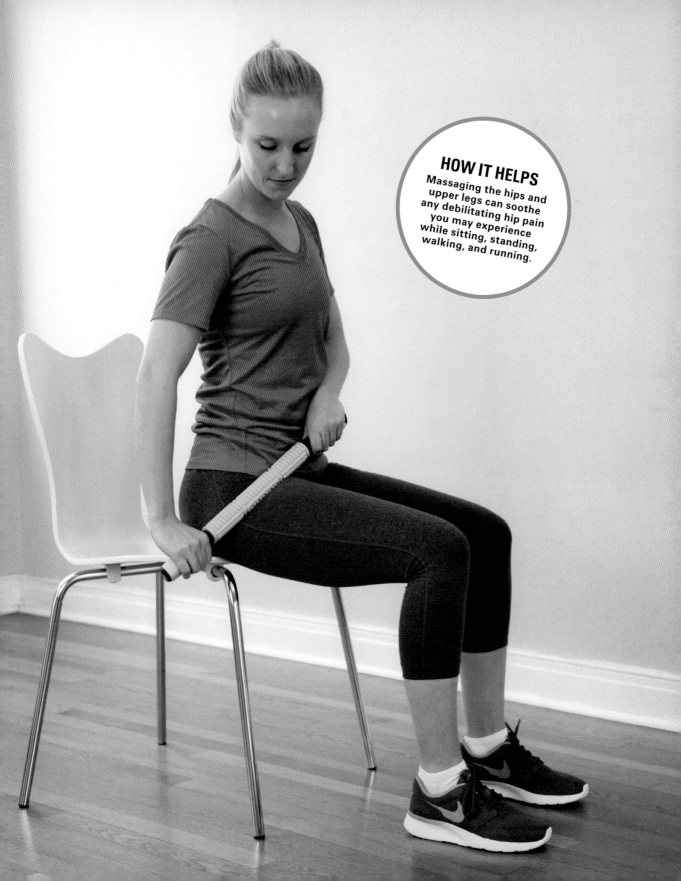

UPPER LEGS

From high-intensity sports to sitting down for long periods, many activities cause knee and hip pain. Disorders of the upper legs often originate from weak or misused muscles. These exercises relieve pain and strengthen the upper legs.

WHAT YOU NEED

- Foam roller
- Massage ball
- Chair
- Yoga mat

WHAT TO DO

- Do the exercises in order.
- Spend 30 to 45 seconds on each exercise.
- Monitor your pain level and adjust the pressure accordingly.
- Maximize soft tissue release by rotating your legs during the exercises.

	EXERCISE	TOOL	PAGE
1	QUADRICEPS RELEASE		P66
2	OUTER THIGH AND HIP RELEASE		P70
3	TARGETED HIP FLEXOR RELEASE		P51
4	TARGETED HAMSTRINGS RELEASE		P74
5	TARGETED INNER THIGH RELEASE		P78
6	CLAMSHELL HIP ROTATION		P56
7	HIP ROTATOR RAISE		P54

QUADRICEPS RELEASE

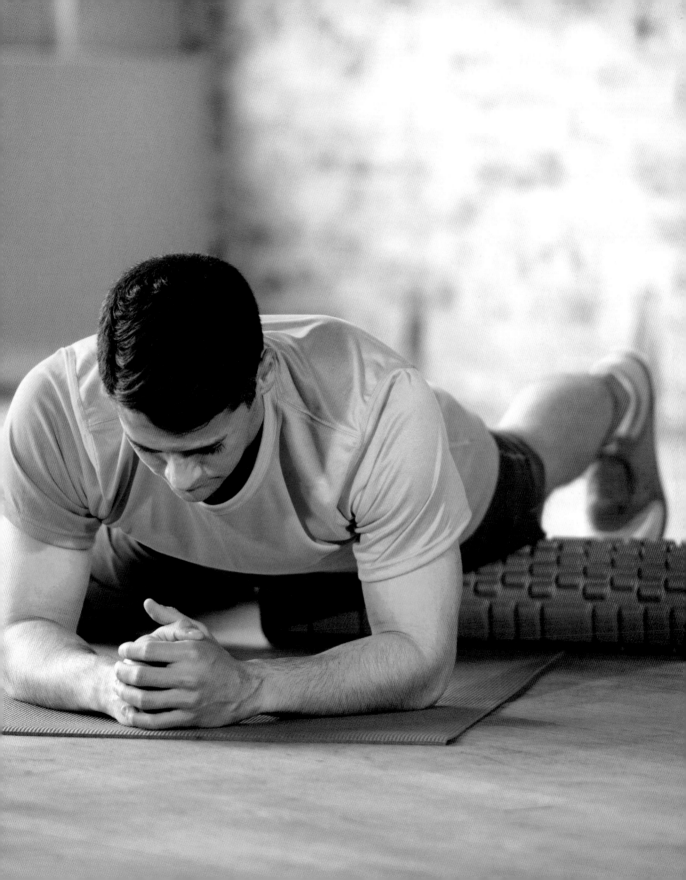

LOWER LEGS

You don't have to be an avid runner to develop lower leg pain – sometimes pressing your car brake and accelerator pedals repeatedly will cause pain. Your lower legs are often overworked, so do these exercises to alleviate discomfort.

WHAT YOU NEED

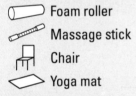

⊐ Foam roller
Massage stick
Chair
Yoga mat

WHAT TO DO

○ Do the exercises in order.
○ Spend 30 to 45 seconds on each exercise.
○ Breathe deeply and relax your muscles.
○ Keep your feet and ankles loose so that your legs are receptive to release.

	EXERCISE	TOOL	PAGE
1	CALF MASSAGE	⊐	P86
2	KNEE RELEASE	⊐	P80
3	SHIN RELEASE	⊐	P82
4	ANKLE RELEASE	⊐	P92
5	ARCH RELEASE		P94

CALF
MASSAGE

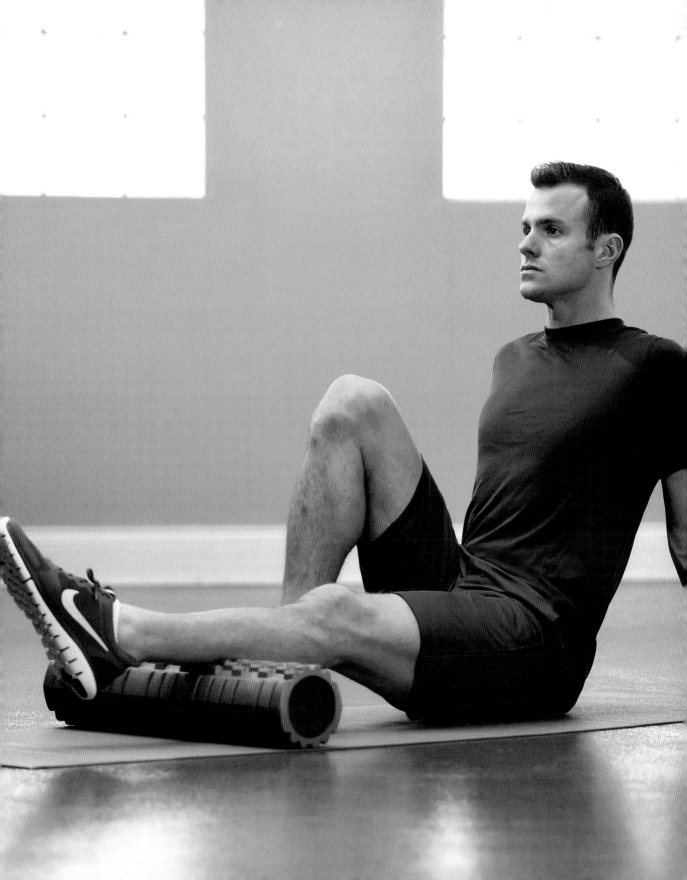

HAND AND FOREARM

As many desk workers, pianists, and tennis players can attest, pain in the forearms and hands can be debilitating in day-to-day activities such as opening a jar or brushing your teeth. Follow this programme to keep pain in your arms at bay.

WHAT YOU NEED

- ◯ Massage ball
- ⬭ Foam roller
- ▱ Yoga mat

WHAT TO DO

- ○ Do the exercises in order.
- ○ Spend 30 to 45 seconds on each exercise.
- ○ Monitor your pain level and adjust the pressure accordingly.
- ○ Relax your hands and wrists.

	EXERCISE	TOOL	PAGE
1	FINGER FLEXOR RELEASE	◯	P**134**
2	FINGER EXTENSOR RELEASE	◯	P**135**
3	TARGETED PALM RELEASE	◯	P**136**
4	TRICEPS RELEASE	⬭	P**128**
5	BICEPS RELEASE	⬭	P**126**
6	CHEST RELEASE	⬭	P**118**

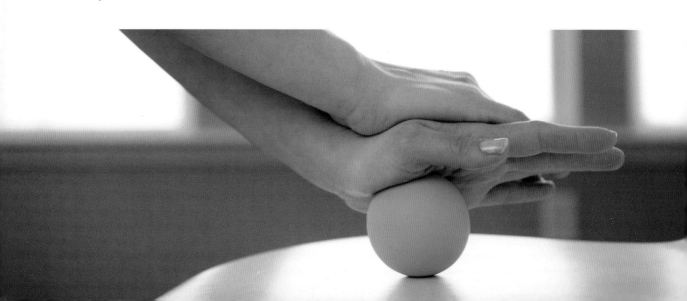

FEET

When you're always wearing socks and shoes, your feet easily become desensitized and painful while diminishing your body awareness. Complete these exercises to prevent or alleviate foot pain and improve your balance.

WHAT YOU NEED

- Massage stick
- Massage ball
- Foam roller
- Half roller
- Chair
- Yoga mat

WHAT TO DO

- Do the exercises in order.
- Spend 30 to 45 seconds on each exercise.
- Breathe deeply and relax your targeted foot.
- Remove your socks and shoes.

	EXERCISE	TOOL	PAGE
1	ARCH RELEASE		P**94**
2	TARGETED CALF RELEASE		P**88**
3	ANKLE RELEASE		P**92**
4	TARGETED FOOT RELEASE		P**95**
5	SPIRAL CALF RAISE		P**90**

HOW IT HELPS

Massaging the soles of your feet sharpens the sensory input from thousands of nerve endings, even when you're wearing shoes.

TARGETED PALM RELEASE

LIFESTYLE PROGRAMMES

TOO MUCH SITTING

Sitting too much is detrimental, as it deteriorates your posture and imbalances your muscles. The result is a myriad of pains and stiff joints throughout your body. Use this programme to counteract the tension and re-establish mobility.

WHAT YOU NEED

- Foam roller
- Half roller
- Yoga mat

WHAT TO DO

- Do the exercises in order.
- Spend 30 to 45 seconds on each exercise.
- Breathe deeply and relax your muscles.
- Use a textured roller for muscles that are especially inhibited.

	EXERCISE	TOOL	PAGE
1	HIP FLEXOR RELEASE		P50
2	QUADRICEPS RELEASE		P66
3	HAMSTRINGS RELEASE		P72
4	SPINE RESTORATION		P98
5	SPINE LENGTHENING		P100
6	GLUTEAL BRIDGE		P62
7	FOREARM WALL SLIDE		P130
8	OVERHEAD SQUAT		P44
9	PLANK PROGRESSIONS		P24

HIP FLEXOR RELEASE

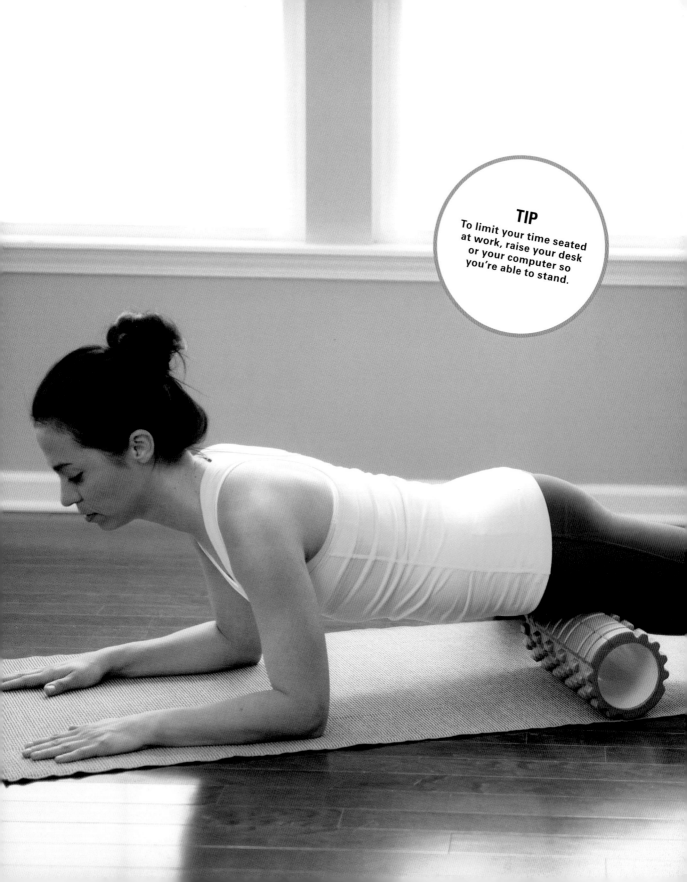

TIP
To limit your time seated at work, raise your desk or your computer so you're able to stand.

TOO MUCH STANDING

Professions that require too much standing, such as restaurant or retail jobs, can freeze your muscles and joints into one position and make them stiff and imbalanced. Do this programme to restore functional movement.

WHAT YOU NEED

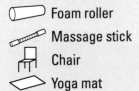

Foam roller
Massage stick
Chair
Yoga mat

WHAT TO DO

- Do the exercises in order.
- Spend 30 to 45 seconds on each exercise.
- Monitor your pain level and adjust the pressure accordingly.
- Remove your shoes for improved body awareness.

EXERCISE	TOOL	PAGE
1 GLUTEAL GROUP RELEASE		P58
2 QUADRICEPS RELEASE		P66
3 HAMSTRINGS RELEASE		P72
4 CALF MASSAGE		P86
5 ARCH RELEASE		P94
6 STRAIGHT-LEG RAISE		P40
7 ROLLER WALKOUT		P28
8 HALF-KNEELING CORE ROTATION		P36
9 STRAIGHT-LEG GLUTEAL BRIDGE		P64

GLUTEAL
GROUP
RELEASE

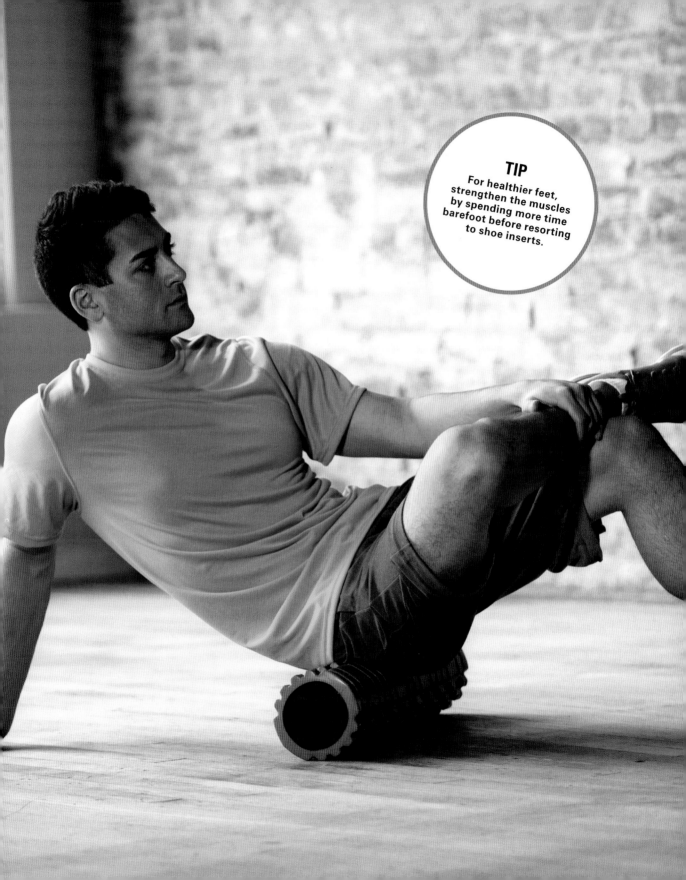

TIP
For healthier feet, strengthen the muscles by spending more time barefoot before resorting to shoe inserts.

ACTIVE LIFESTYLE

Walking a dog, gardening, or taking care of children all require mobility in several key areas of your body, and core stability to protect your spine. Perform this programme regularly to support the dynamic movements of your active lifestyle.

WHAT YOU NEED

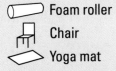

Foam roller

Chair

Yoga mat

WHAT TO DO

- Do the exercises in order.
- Spend 30 to 45 seconds on each exercise.
- Breathe deeply and relax your muscles.
- Modify the exercise or go to the next one if it's too difficult to maintain perfect posture.

	EXERCISE	TOOL	PAGE
1	SPINE RESTORATION		P98
2	LATS RELEASE		P122
3	BIRD DOG REACH		P30
4	SPINE LENGTHENING		P100
5	FOREARM WALL SLIDE		P130
6	ADDUCTOR CHAIR SQUAT		P48
7	PLANK PROGRESSIONS		P24
8	SITTING RIBCAGE ROTATION		P34

ADDUCTOR CHAIR SQUAT

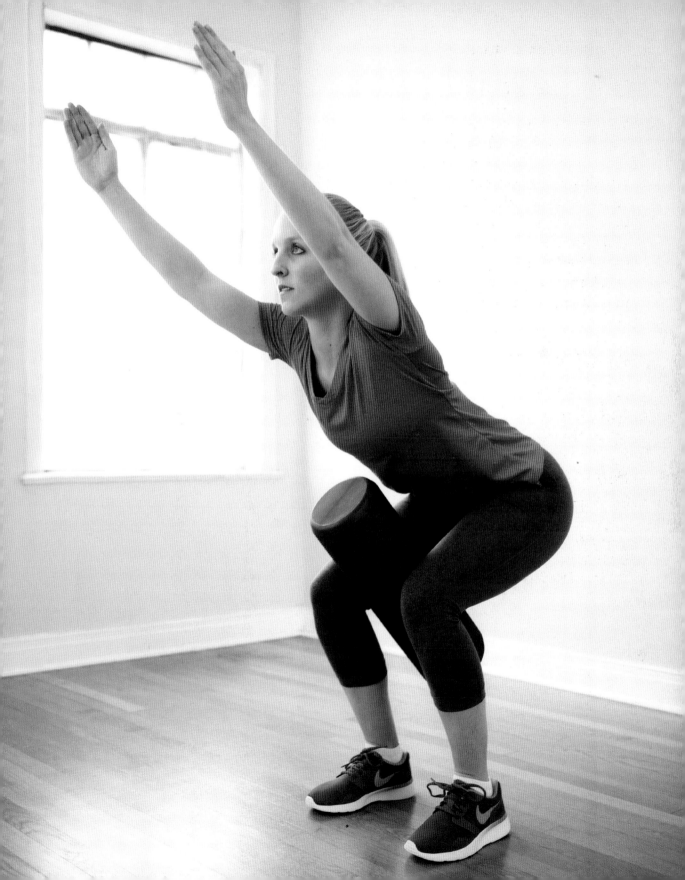

DAILY CONDITIONING

Massaging your muscles and doing rotational exercises on a daily basis will make your body feel more awake and capable during day-to-day movements. Follow this easy programme to prime your body for a productive day.

WHAT YOU NEED

- ◯ Massage ball
- ⬭ Full roller
- ▱ Yoga mat

WHAT TO DO

- o Do the exercises in order.
- o Spend 30 to 45 seconds on each exercise.
- o Monitor your pain level and adjust the pressure accordingly.
- o Breathe deeply to relax your body.

	EXERCISE	TOOL	PAGE
1	TARGETED FOOT RELEASE	◯	P95
2	OUTER THIGH AND HIP RELEASE	⬭	P70
3	INNER THIGH RELEASE	⬭	P76
4	SPINE RESTORATION	⬭	P98
5	SIDE-LYING RIBCAGE ROTATION	⬭	P38
6	HIP SWIVEL	⬭	P32

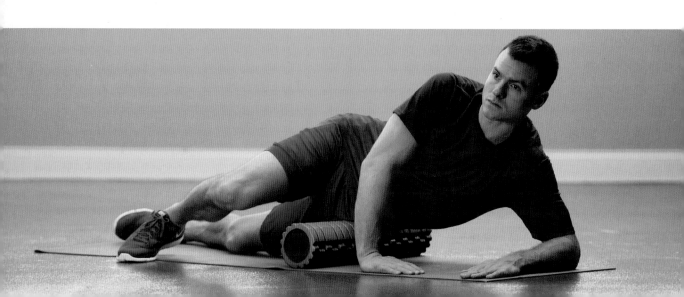

OVERHEAD REACHING RELIEF

Cleaning a window, stacking a shelf, and writing on a white- or blackboard easily overworks and strains your arms and shoulders. If you have to reach overhead often, complete these exercises to loosen the muscles and prevent injury.

WHAT YOU NEED

- Foam roller
- Massage ball
- Massage stick
- Yoga mat

WHAT TO DO

- Do the exercises in order.
- Spend 30 to 45 seconds on each exercise.
- Breathe deeply and relax your muscles.
- Monitor the pain level in your shoulders, and adjust the pressure accordingly.

	EXERCISE	TOOL	PAGE
1	SPINE RESTORATION		P98
2	TARGETED SHOULDER RELEASE		P112
3	LATS RELEASE		P122
4	NECK RELEASE		P132
5	TARGETED MIDDLE BACK RELEASE		P108
6	SHOULDER BLADE MOBILIZATION		P116
7	SPINE LENGTHENING		P100

OUTER THIGH AND HIP RELEASE

POSTURE RESTORATION

Anything from tightly fitting clothing to bucket seats in a car can contribute to poor posture. Even sports such as rowing and cycling are detrimental to spine health. Perform these exercises regularly to restore your alignment.

WHAT YOU NEED

- Foam roller
- Half roller
- Yoga mat

WHAT TO DO

- Do the exercises in order.
- Spend 30 to 45 seconds on each exercise.
- Monitor your pain level and adjust the pressure accordingly.
- Modify any exercise that becomes too easy, or increase your repetitions.

	EXERCISE	TOOL	PAGE
1	SPINE RESTORATION		P98
2	SPINE LENGTHENING		P100
3	LATS RELEASE		P122
4	FOREARM WALL SLIDE		P130
5	QUADRICEPS RELEASE		P66
6	GLUTEAL BRIDGE		P62
7	ROLLER ROLLOUT		P26
8	STRAIGHT-LEG RAISE		P40
9	OVERHEAD SQUAT		P44

LATS RELEASE ▶

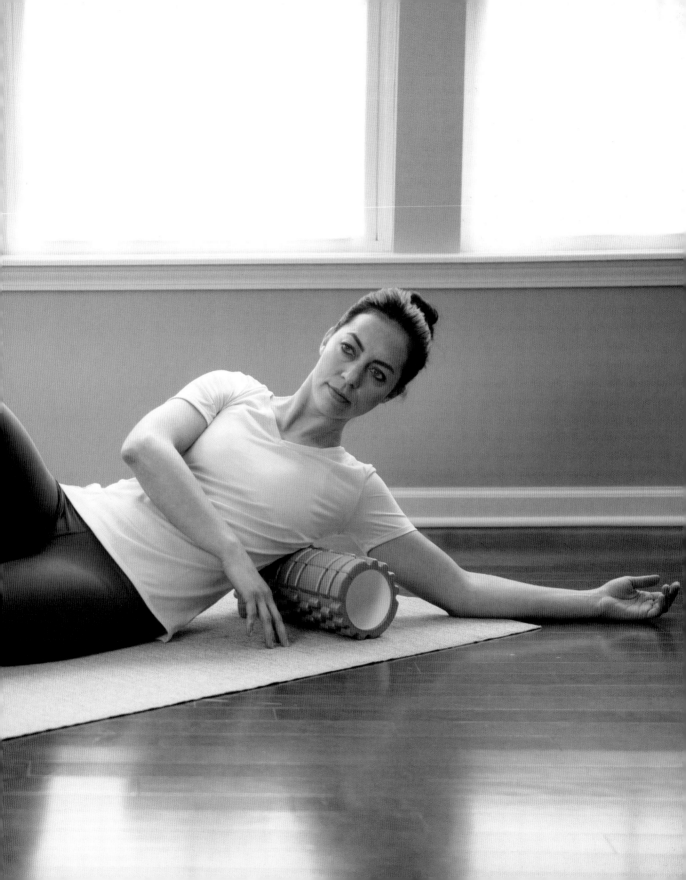

STRESS RELIEF

Whatever the stresses in your life, they often translate into muscle tension. The exercises in this programme will release the areas where you may tend to carry the most pressure so your body can feel lighter, looser, and pain-free.

WHAT YOU NEED

◯ Massage ball
⬭ Massage stick
▭ Foam roller
▱ Yoga mat

WHAT TO DO

- Do the exercises in order.
- Spend 30 to 45 seconds on each exercise.
- Breathe deeply and relax your muscles.
- Set aside 10 minutes for the exercises in a quiet, distraction-free environment.

	EXERCISE	TOOL	PAGE
1	**TARGETED PALM RELEASE**	◯	P136
2	**NECK RELEASE**	⬭	P132
3	**TARGETED SHOULDER RELEASE**	◯	P112
4	**TARGETED MIDDLE BACK RELEASE**	◯	P108
5	**TARGETED HIP ROTATOR RELEASE**	◯	P52
6	**TARGETED FOOT RELEASE**	◯	P95
7	**SPINE LENGTHENING**	▭	P100

LIMITED MOBILITY

Joints conform to the positions in which you most frequently hold them, so if you're in one position for extended periods, your joints can lose mobility. Perform these exercises to counteract the most commonly stiff joints in your body.

WHAT YOU NEED

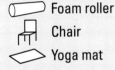

Foam roller

Chair

Yoga mat

WHAT TO DO

- Do the exercises in order.
- Spend 30 to 45 seconds on each exercise.
- Monitor your pain level and adjust the pressure accordingly.
- Modify the exercise if it's difficult to maintain good posture.

EXERCISE	TOOL	PAGE
1 HIP FLEXOR RELEASE		P**50**
2 QUADRICEPS RELEASE		P**66**
3 SPINE RESTORATION		P**98**
4 FOREARM WALL SLIDE		P**130**
5 ROLLER WALKOUT		P**28**
6 SITTING RIBCAGE ROTATION		P**34**
7 HALF-KNEELING CORE ROTATION		P**36**

HOW IT HELPS

Foam rolling the muscle around your joints breaks up adhesions from injury and improves flexibility.

FULL BODY RELAXATION

This programme is perfect for the end of the day when you need to relax. It's only five exercises, so spend extra time on those that feel best. With slow, deep breathing, you'll feel the tension melt away after completing the exercise.

WHAT YOU NEED

- Massage ball
- Foam roller
- Massage stick
- Yoga mat

WHAT TO DO

- Do the exercises in order.
- Spend 30 to 45 seconds on each exercise.
- Breathe deeply and relax your muscles.
- Remove distractions from the area and allow your muscles to melt over the tools.

	EXERCISE	TOOL	PAGE
1	TARGETED LOWER BACK RELEASE		P104
2	MIDDLE BACK RELEASE		P106
3	SPINE RESTORATION		P98
4	SPINE LENGTHENING		P100
5	NECK RELEASE		P132

HOW IT HELPS

When you ease muscle tension, your heart rate slows, your breathing relaxes, and your body begins to heal.

TARGETED LOWER BACK RELEASE

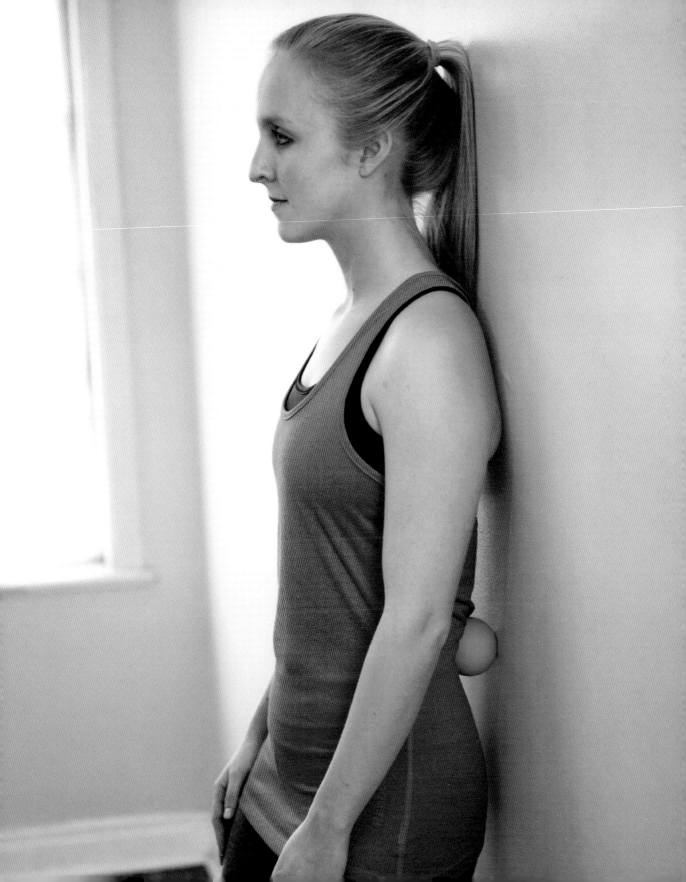

WEEKEND WARRIOR

If you're a desk worker during the week but a warrior at the weekend, do this programme to complement your ambitious fitness endeavours. This well-rounded routine awakens the muscles before a workout, or do it briskly as your main workout.

WHAT YOU NEED

- ○ Massage ball
- ⬭ Foam roller
- ◇ Yoga mat

WHAT TO DO

- ○ Do the exercises in order.
- ○ Spend 30 to 45 seconds on each exercise.
- ○ Breathe deeply and relax your muscles.
- ○ Remove your shoes for the first exercise to improve balance for the remaining ones.

	EXERCISE	TOOL	PAGE
1	TARGETED FOOT RELEASE	○	P95
2	SPINE RESTORATION	⬭	P98
3	HIP FLEXOR RELEASE	⬭	P50
4	GLUTEAL BRIDGE	⬭	P62
5	CLAMSHELL HIP ROTATION	⬭	P56
6	STRAIGHT-LEG RAISE	⬭	P40
7	BIRD DOG REACH	⬭	P30
8	HIP SWIVEL	⬭	P32
9	ADDUCTOR CHAIR SQUAT	⬭	P48

TARGETED FOOT RELEASE

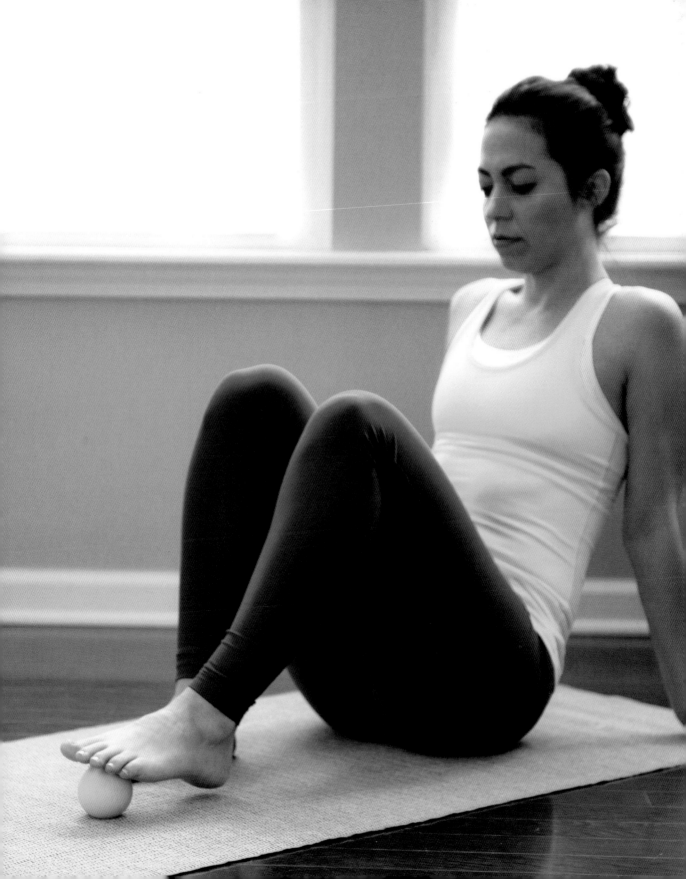

LIFETIME MOBILITY

With age, mobility can gradually diminish. Make a point of foam rolling your muscles often to lessen your chances of sustaining mobility-related injuries. These exercises keep muscles flexible and your body awareness high.

WHAT YOU NEED

Foam roller

Massage ball

Yoga mat

WHAT TO DO

o Do the exercises in order.

o Spend 30 to 45 seconds on each exercise.

o Monitor your pain level and adjust the pressure accordingly.

o Perform the exercise against a wall or in a chair when it's difficult to get into position.

	EXERCISE	TOOL	PAGE
1	CHEST RELEASE		P118
2	MIDDLE BACK ACTIVATION		P110
3	TARGETED HIP FLEXOR RELEASE		P51
4	TARGETED SHIN RELEASE		P84
5	BIRD DOG REACH		P30
6	TARGETED FOOT RELEASE		P95

TIP

For healthy ageing and strength, it's important to stay active. Exercise significantly reduces the risk of diminished mobility.

PAIN MANAGEMENT

The stresses of your life can sometimes be enough to produce aches and knots that refer pain through your whole body. If you feel an overall ache in your joints and muscles, do this programme to tackle common areas of tightness.

WHAT YOU NEED

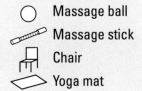

○ Massage ball

Massage stick

Chair

Yoga mat

WHAT TO DO

- Do the exercises in order.
- Spend 30 to 45 seconds on each exercise.
- Breathe deeply and relax your muscles.
- Increase or decrease pressure to maintain a productive level of discomfort.

	EXERCISE	TOOL	PAGE
1	TARGETED PALM RELEASE	○	P**136**
2	NECK RELEASE	(massage stick)	P**132**
3	TARGETED CHEST RELEASE	○	P**120**
4	TARGETED SHOULDER RELEASE	○	P**112**
5	TARGETED MIDDLE BACK RELEASE	○	P**108**
6	TARGETED HAMSTRINGS RELEASE	○	P**74**
7	TARGETED GLUTEAL GROUP RELEASE	○	P**60**
8	TARGETED QUADRICEPS RELEASE	○	P**68**
9	TARGETED CALF RELEASE	○	P**88**
10	TARGETED FOOT RELEASE	○	P**95**

SPORTS
PROGRAMMES

PRE-WORKOUT

To provide a dynamic warm-up for your muscles, a routine should include as much foam rolling as possible in addition to challenging, active movements. Complete these exercises to loosen your muscles for an injury-free workout.

WHAT YOU NEED

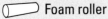 Foam roller

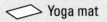 Half roller

Yoga mat

WHAT TO DO

- Do the exercises in order.
- Spend 30 to 45 seconds on each exercise.
- Breathe deeply and relax your muscles.
- Maintain a moderate pace for exercises 5 to 8 to accelerate your circulation.

	EXERCISE	TOOL	PAGE
1	GLUTEAL GROUP RELEASE		P58
2	QUADRICEPS RELEASE		P66
3	OUTER THIGH AND HIP RELEASE		P70
4	SPINE RESTORATION		P98
5	STRAIGHT-LEG RAISE		P40
6	STRAIGHT-LEG GLUTEAL BRIDGE		P64
7	ROLLER ROLLOUT		P26
8	OVERHEAD SQUAT		P44

HOW IT HELPS
Warming up gently increases your heart rate to loosen joints and increase the blood flow to muscles.

STRAIGHT-LEG RAISE

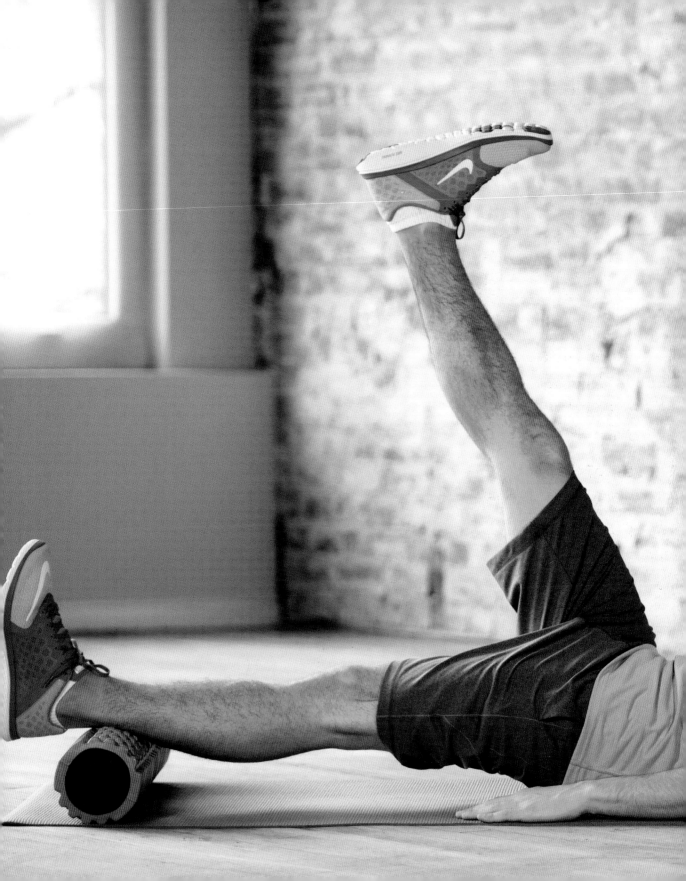

POST-WORKOUT

After any kind of workout, your body needs time to slow the heart rate and maximize gains in the range of movement of the muscles. Do this programme to restore a comfortable breathing pattern and to ensure post-workout flexibility.

WHAT YOU NEED

Foam roller

Yoga mat

WHAT TO DO

- Do the exercises in order.
- Spend 30 to 45 seconds on each exercise.
- Breathe deeply and relax your muscles.
- Repeat the programme if your heart rate is still rapid after the first completion.

	EXERCISE	TOOL	PAGE
1	ROLLER WALKOUT		P28
2	SIDE-LYING RIBCAGE ROTATION		P38
3	BIRD DOG REACH		P30
4	HIP SWIVEL		P32
5	HALF-KNEELING RIBCAGE ROTATION		P36

ROLLER WALKOUT ▶

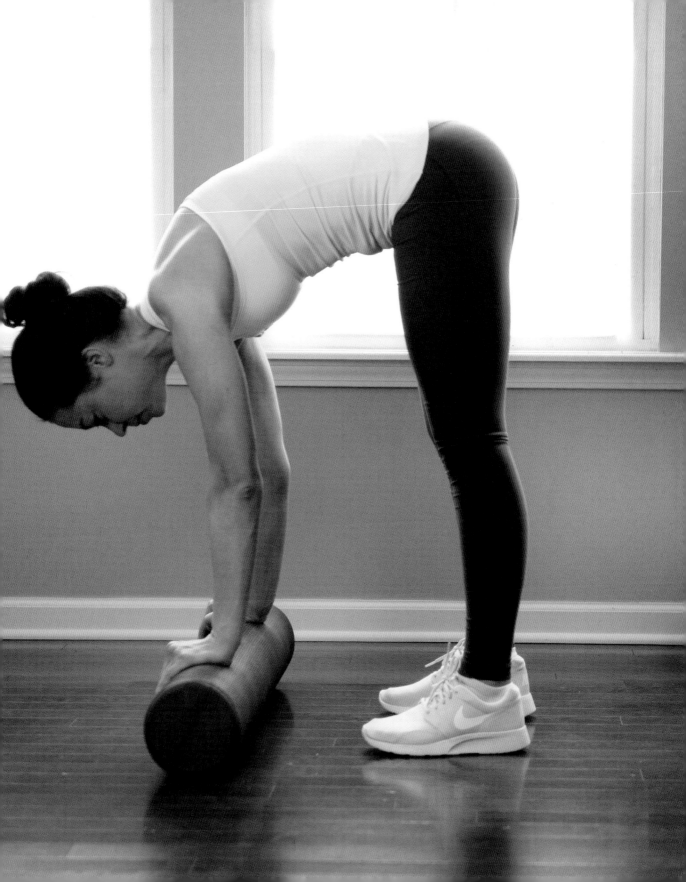

STRAIGHT-LINE SPORTS

"Straight-line" sports such as skiing and running require core stability and healthy mobility in the ankles, hips, and thoracic spine. Complete this programme to reinforce core and lower body coordination for a more functional forward motion.

WHAT YOU NEED

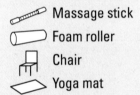

Massage stick
Foam roller
Chair
Yoga mat

WHAT TO DO

- Do the exercises in order.
- Spend 30 to 45 seconds on each exercise.
- Breathe deeply and relax your muscles.
- Modify any exercise that becomes too easy, or increase your repetitions.

	EXERCISE	TOOL	PAGE
1	ARCH RELEASE		P94
2	INNER THIGH RELEASE		P76
3	OUTER THIGH AND HIP RELEASE		P70
4	CLAMSHELL HIP ROTATION		P56
5	STRAIGHT-LEG RAISE		P40
6	ROLLER WALKOUT		P28
7	HALF-KNEELING CORE ROTATION		P36
8	PLANK PROGRESSIONS		P24

HALF-KNEELING CORE ROTATION ▶

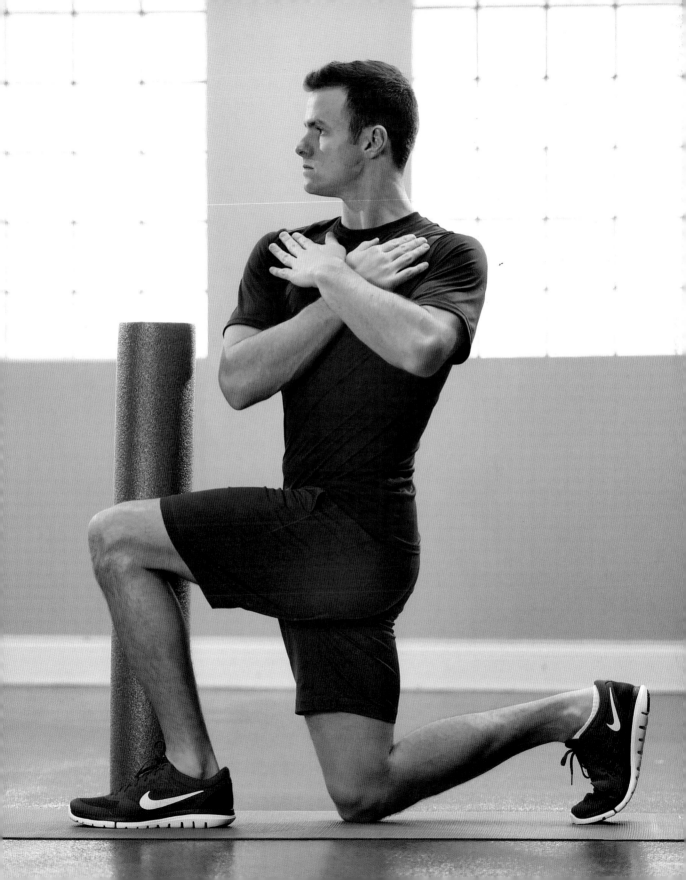

ROTATIONAL SPORTS

Sports such as tennis, squash, golf, and cricket demand the ability to coordinate torso rotation with lower body movement. Do these exercises to improve your balance and stability during movements such as swinging a racquet.

WHAT YOU NEED

- ◯ Massage ball
- ▭ Foam roller
- ◣ Half roller
- ▱ Yoga mat

WHAT TO DO

- ○ Do the exercises in order.
- ○ Spend 30 to 45 seconds on each exercise.
- ○ Breathe deeply and lengthen your torso.
- ○ Remove your shoes for the first exercise to improve your balance for the remaining exercises in the programme.

	EXERCISE	TOOL	PAGE
1	TARGETED FOOT RELEASE	◯	P95
2	SPINE RESTORATION	▭	P98
3	LATS RELEASE	▭	P122
4	SPIRAL CALF RAISE	◣◯	P90
5	BIRD DOG REACH	▭	P30
6	HIP SWIVEL	▭	P32
7	PLANK PROGRESSIONS	▭	P24
8	ROTATIONAL LUNGE	▭	P46

ROTATIONAL LUNGE ▶

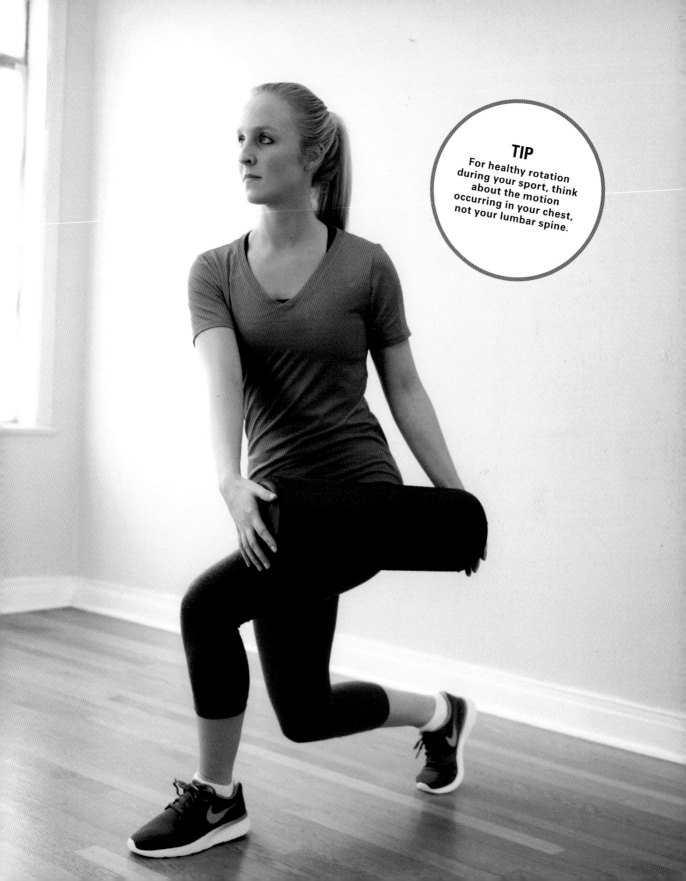

TIP
For healthy rotation during your sport, think about the motion occurring in your chest, not your lumbar spine.

OVERHEAD SPORTS

Overhead sports such as swimming and volleyball require strong and flexible shoulder joints and upper body muscles to safely perform the reaching movements. Do these exercises to improve the mobility of your shoulder complex.

WHAT YOU NEED

- Foam roller
- Half roller
- Yoga mat

WHAT TO DO

- Do the exercises in order.
- Spend 30 to 45 seconds on each exercise.
- Breathe deeply and relax your muscles.
- Perform additional repetitions if an exercise becomes too easy.

	EXERCISE	TOOL	PAGE
1	SPINE RESTORATION		P98
2	LATS RELEASE		P122
3	MIDDLE BACK ACTIVATION		P110
4	SHOULDER BLADE MOBILIZATION		P116
5	FRONT SHOULDER RELEASE		P115
6	FOREARM WALL SLIDE		P130
7	ROLLER ROLLOUT		P26
8	OVERHEAD SQUAT		P44

OVERHEAD SQUAT

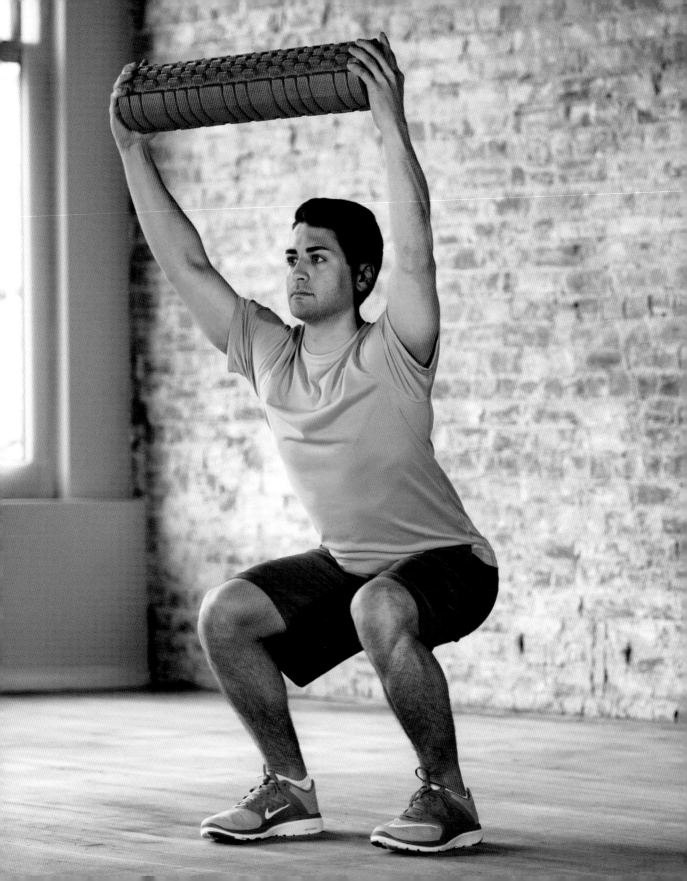

INDEX

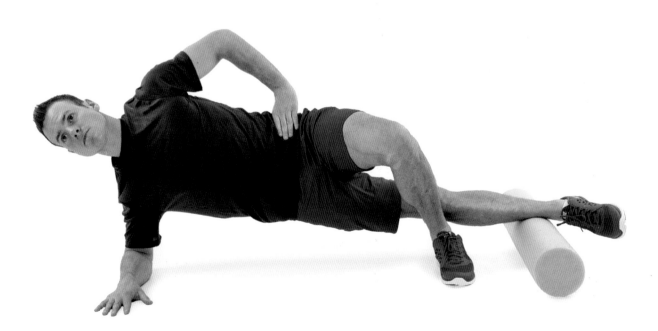

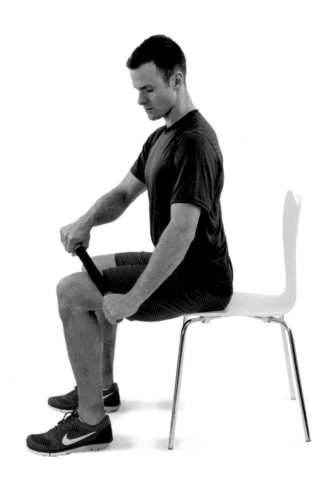

ABOUT THE AUTHOR

Sam Woodworth is a personal trainer with a degree in Exercise science from Ball State University in the US. He is a certified Level 2 Functional movement systems professional and a Level 2 EBFA barefoot training specialist. Sam strives to keep people pain-free by identifying occupational and recreational obstacles and ensuring they have the tools for healthy movement. As a trainer, Sam uses foam rollers and other myofascial release equipment with clients to improve mobility and stability, ease pain, and promote recovery. Contact Sam for further information and for answers to any questions about functional movement by visiting his website: samwoodworth-trainer.com.

ACKNOWLEDGEMENTS

First and foremost, thank you to my mum, Karen Woodworth. You are without a doubt the most influential person in my life, and I owe everything to your hard work and unconditional love. Thank you also to Art Brock and Teresa Rogers for giving me the opportunity six years ago to help others and to come into my own as I do what I love. Lastly, thank you to my editor, Ann Barton: you've undoubtedly changed my life for the better by giving me this opportunity to positively affect people's lives on a big scale. Thank you, all!

PUBLISHER'S ACKNOWLEDGEMENTS

The publisher would like to thank Sam Woodworth, Niki Waddell, Cort Post, and Olga Alkhutova for their modelling talent.

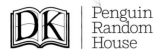

DK UK
Angliciser: Susannah Steel
Project Editor: Kathryn Meeker
Senior Art Editor: Glenda Fisher
Assistant Designer: Philippa Nash
Jacket Designer: Harriet Yeomans
Pre-production Producer: Robert Dunn
Senior Producer: Stephanie McConnell
Creative Technical Support: Sonia Charbonnier
Managing Editor: Stephanie Farrow
Senior Managing Art Editor: Christine Keilty

DK USA
Publisher: Mike Sanders
Associate Publisher: Billy Fields
Acquisitions Editor: Ann Barton
Development Editor: Alexandra Elliott
Book Designer: XAB Design
Photographer: Matt Bowen
Art Director for Photography: XAB Design
Prepress Technician: Brian Massey
Proofreader: Amy Borrelli
Indexer: Brad Herriman

First published in Great Britain in 2017 by
Dorling Kindersley Limited
80 Strand, London, WC2R 0RL

Copyright © 2017 Dorling Kindersley Limited
A Penguin Random House Company
10 9 8 7 6 5 4 3 2 1
001–296974–Jan/2017

A CIP catalogue record for this book
is available from the British Library.
ISBN: 978-0-2412-7531-3

Printed and bound in China

All images © Dorling Kindersley Limited
For further information see: www.dkimages.com

A WORLD OF IDEAS:
SEE ALL THERE IS TO KNOW

www.dk.com